Ammar Hadi
Jamal Faraj
Ala Abass

Rehabilitation of Chronic Obstructive Pulmonary Disease

Ammar Hadi
Jamal Faraj
Ala Abass

Rehabilitation of Chronic Obstructive Pulmonary Disease

Noor Publishing

Imprint

Any brand names and product names mentioned in this book are subject to trademark, brand or patent protection and are trademarks or registered trademarks of their respective holders. The use of brand names, product names, common names, trade names, product descriptions etc. even without a particular marking in this work is in no way to be construed to mean that such names may be regarded as unrestricted in respect of trademark and brand protection legislation and could thus be used by anyone.

Cover image: www.ingimage.com

Publisher:
Noor Publishing
is a trademark of
International Book Market Service Ltd., member of OmniScriptum Publishing Group
17 Meldrum Street, Beau Bassin 71504, Mauritius

Printed at: see last page
ISBN: 978-620-0-06370-0

Zugl. / Approved by: Babylon, University of Babylon, {May}., 2019

REHABILITATION

Of

CHRONIC OBSTRUCTIVE PULMONARY DISEASE

A GUIDE TO YOUR TREATMENT

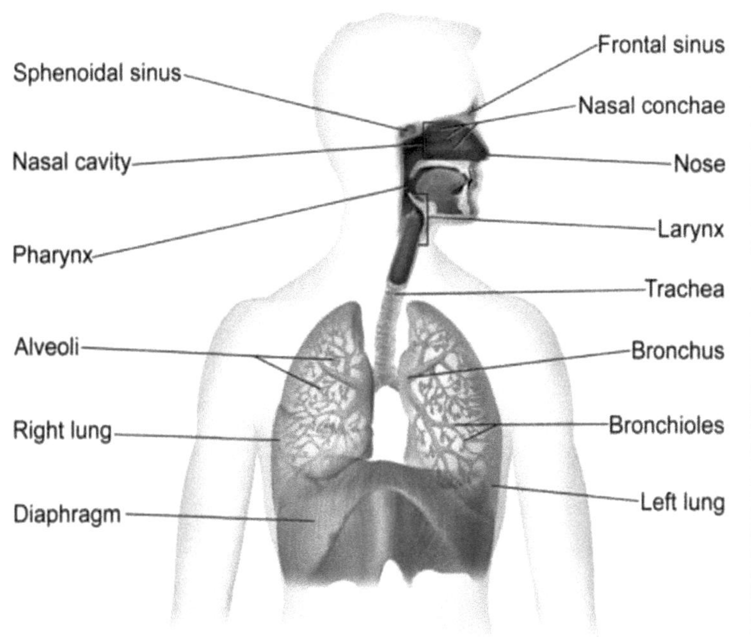

Prof. Dr Ammar Hamza Hadi

Prof. Dr Jamal Sabri Faraj

Prof. Dr Ala Hussain Abass

REHABILITATION

Of

CHRONIC OBSTRUCTIVE PULMONARY DISEASE

A GUIDE TO YOUR TREATMENT

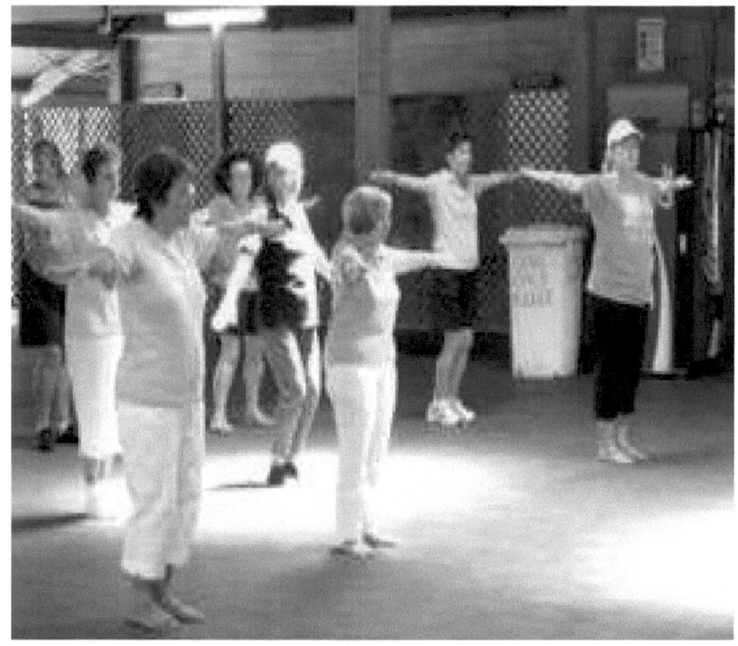

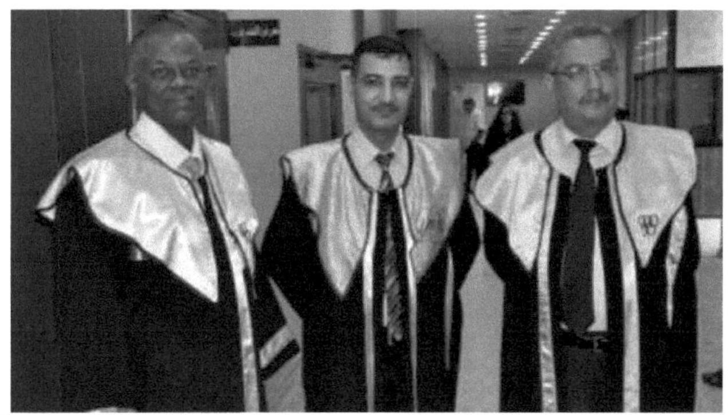

Each year, we learn more about rehabilitation benefits of staying physically active and being properly nourished throughout our lives. The work of scientists, rehabilitation professionals, and older adult volunteers have greatly increased our knowledge about the chronic obstructive pulmonary disease rehabilitation process and how we can maintain strength, endurance, dignity, and independence as we age.

Essential to treatment chronic obstructive pulmonary disease patients and staying healthy and vital during older adulthood is participation in regular rehabilitation exercises, which help to improve quality of life, reduce morbidity and mortality, and prevent increasing of severity of disease. Feeling physically strong also promotes mental and emotional health. Rehabilitation exercises are easy to learn, and have been proven safe and effective through years of thorough research.

Experts at the Morjan Hospital for Disease Control and Prevention and Babylon University, with the help of older adults, have created this book, ***REHABILITATION Of CHRONIC OBSTRUCTIVE PULMONARY DISEASE*** to help you become healthy and maintain your respiratory system and independence. We encourage you to read it carefully and begin using this rehabilitation programs as soon as possible. It can make a profound difference in your physical, mental, emotional health, and quality of life.

Authors

REHABILITATION

Of

CHRONIC OBSTRUCTIVE PULMONARY DISEASE

A GUIDE TO YOUR TREATMENT

Ammar H. H. Prof. PhD [1]

Jamal S. F., Prof. PhD [2]

Ala H. A., Prof. PhD [3]

[1] Health Sciences Group/ Physical Education & Sport Sciences Faculty/ Babylon University.

[2] Sport Training Group/ Physical Education & Sport Sciences Faculty/ Babylon University. Member of Arab Sport Sciences.

[3] Head of Medical Department/ College of Medicine/ Babylon University..

Contents

Chapter One

Anatomy and Histology of Respiratory System

Anatomy of Respiratory System

The respiratory system divides into an upper and a lower respiratory system (Fig. 1) the upper respiratory system consists of the nose, nasal cavity, paranasal sinuses, and pharynx. These passageways filter, warm, and humidity the incoming air protecting the more delicate surfaces of the lower respiratory system and cool and dehumidify outgoing air. The lower respiratory system includes the larynx (voice box), trachea (windpipe), bronchi, bronchioles, and alveoli of the lungs.

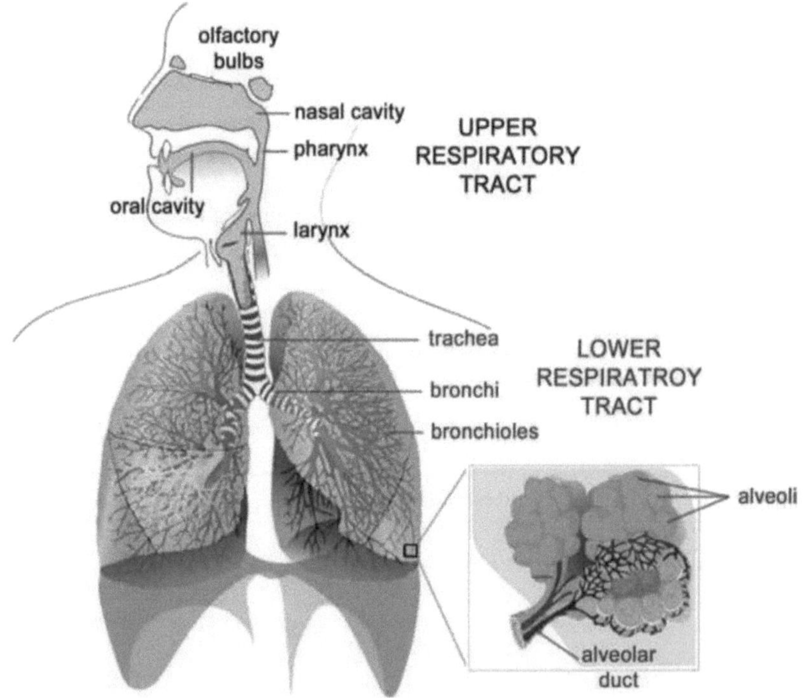

Fig. 1 The components of the respirator system

The Nose and Nasal Cavity

The human nose differs in its anatomy and morphology between different racial and ethnic groups. Therefore, the following anatomical description is a generalization and inter-racial variations exist. For completeness, structures that have synonyms are followed by their alternate names in parentheses and italicised. Structurally the nose is the primary passageway for air entering the respiratory system and it is the only noticeable part of the respiratory system, protruding from the face, and lying in between the forehead and the upper lip. It is made up of a bony section and a cartilaginous section. The bony section is located in the superior half and contains a pair of nasal bones sitting together side by side, separated in the middle and fused posteriorly by the medial plates of the cheekbones (maxilla bones) (Fig. 2). The cartilaginous section is located in the inferior half, consisting of flexible cartilages in the anterior, caudal portion of the nose (Fig. 3). The cartilages are connected to each other and to the bones by a tough fibrous membrane.

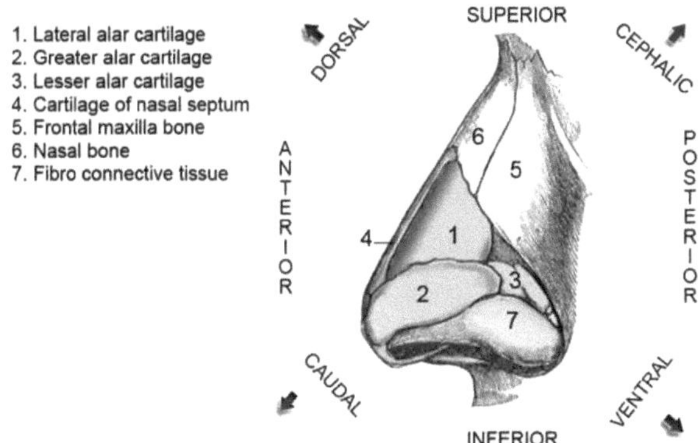

Fig. 2 Lateral view of the external nose showing the cartilage and bone structure. Terminology for the anatomical directions is also given

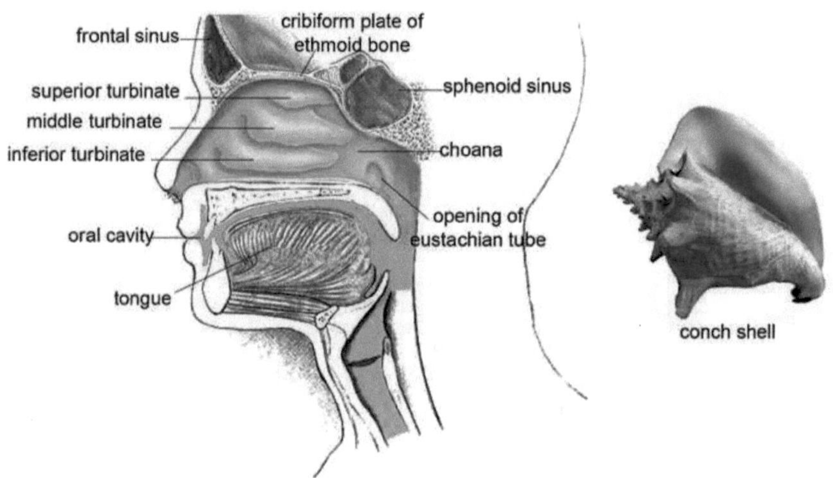

Fig. 3 Structure of the internal nasal cavity. The turbinates are also referred to as concha because of its resemblance to a conch shell

Air normally enters through the paired external nares, or nostrils (Fig. 4), which open into the nasal cavity. The vestibule is the space contained within the flexible tissues of the nose. The epithelium of the vestibule contains coarse hairs that extend across the external nares. Large airborne particles, such as sand, sawdust, or even insects, are trapped in these hairs and are thereby prevented from entering the nasal cavity.

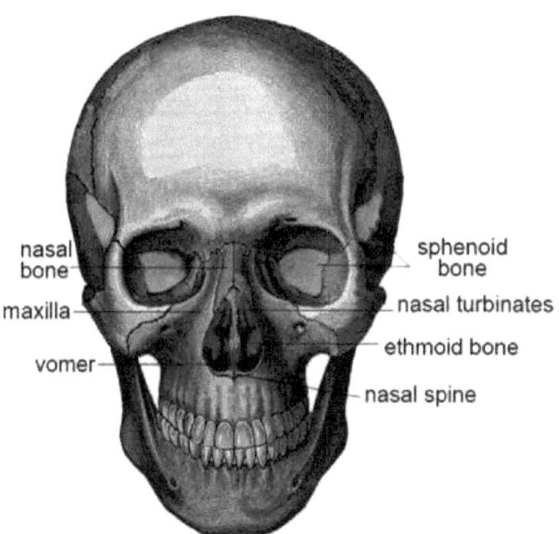

Fig. 4 Skeletal structure of the human skull showing the nasal cavity and the supporting facial bones

The nasal septum divides the nasal cavity into left and right portions (Fig. 5). The bony portion of the nasal septum is formed by the fusion of the perpendicular plate of the ethmoid bone and the plate of the vomer. The anterior portion of the nasal septum is formed of hyaline cartilage. This cartilaginous plate supports the dorsum nasi, or bridge, and apex (tip) of the nose.

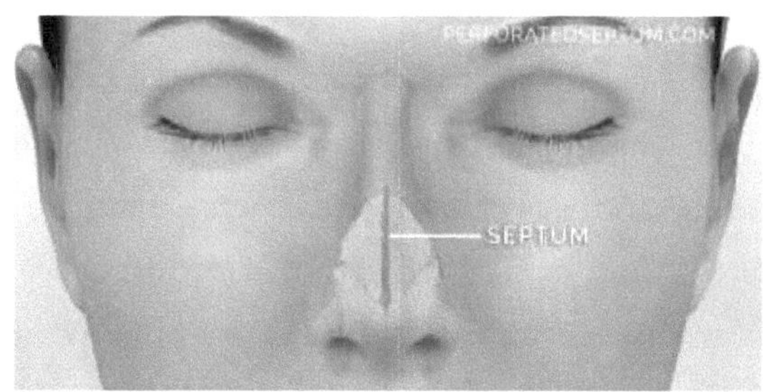

Fig. 5 Shows nasal septum

The maxillary, nasal, frontal, ethmoid, and sphenoid bones form the lateral and superior walls of the nasal cavity. The mucous secretion produced in the associated paranasal sinuses, aided by the tears draining through the nasolacrimal ducts, help keep the surface of the nasal cavity moist and clean. The paranasal sinuses are four pairs of empty air spaces that open or drain into the nasal cavity. They are located in the frontal, sphenoid, ethmoid, and maxillary bones and as such their names are taken from where they are located. The frontal sinuses are located just above the orbit (eye sockets) and don't develop until around the age of seven. The maxillary, the largest of the sinuses extends laterally (into the maxilla) on either side of the nose and is present at birth and grows with the body's development. The sphenoid sinuses lie in the body of the sphenoid bone, deep in the face just behind the nose. This sinus does not develop until adolescence. The ethmoid sinuses are not single large cavities but rather a collection of small air pockets, located around the area of the bridge of the nose. This sinus is also present at birth, and grows with development.

The olfactory region, or superior portion of the nasal cavity, includes the areas lined by olfactory epithelium: (1) the inferior surface of the cribriform plate, (2) the superior portion of the nasal septum, and (3) the superior nasal conchae. Receptors in the olfactory epithelium provide your sense of smell.

The superior, middle, and inferior nasal conchae project toward the nasal septum from the lateral walls of the nasal cavity. To pass from the vestibule to the internal nares, air tends to flow between adjacent conchae, through the superior, middle, and inferior meatuses. These are narrow grooves rather than open passageways; the incoming air bounces off the conchal surfaces and churns like a stream flowing over rapids. This turbulence serves a purpose: As the air eddies and swirls, small airborne particles are likely to come into contact with the mucus that coats the lining of the nasal cavity. In addition to promoting filtration, the turbulence allows extra time for warming and humidifying incoming air. It also creates eddy currents that bring olfactory stimuli to the olfactory receptors.

A bony hard palate made up of portions of the maxillary and palatine bones, forms the floor of the nasal cavity and separates it from the oral cavity. A fleshy soft palate extends posterior to the hard palate, marking the boundary between the superior nasopharynx and the rest of the pharynx. The nasal cavity opens into the nasopharynx through a connection knows as the internal nares.

The Pharynx

The pharynx (throat) is a chamber shared by the digestive and respiratory system. Structure about 12.5 cm long that connects the posterior nasal and oral cavities to the larynx and oesophagus. It extends from the base of the skull to the level of the sixth cervical vertebrae. Structurally the pharynx can be divided into three anatomical parts according to its location as shown in Fig. 6, which are the nasopharynx (posterior to the nasal chambers), the oropharynx (posterior to the mouth), and the laryngopharynx (posterior to the pharynx).

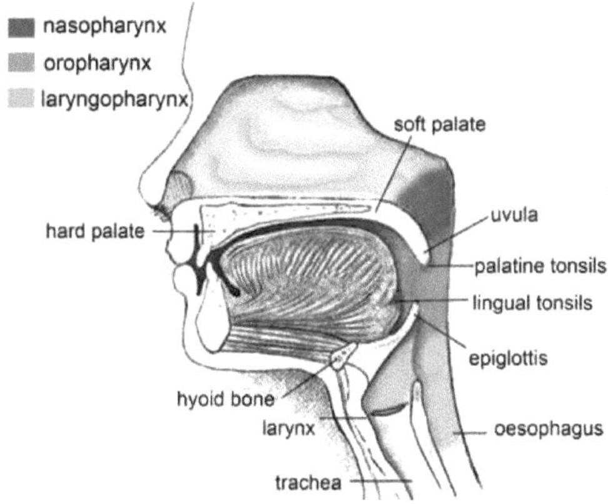

Fig. 6 The pharynx and its subdivisions into the nasopharynx, oropharynx, and laryngopharynx

1. The **nasopharynx** is the superior portion of the pharynx. It is located between the internal nares and the soft palate and lies superior to the oral cavity. At the base of the nasopharynx are the soft palate and the uvula. At the wall of the nasopharynx are the auditory (Eustachian) tubes connected to the middle ear. The pharyngeal tonsils (adenoids) are located in the nasopharynx on its posterior wall opposite the posterior internal nares.

2. The **oropharynx** is located posterior to the mouth, inferior from the soft palate, and superior to the level of the hyoid bone. At this location the mouth leads into the oropharynx and both food and inhaled air pass through it. The palatine (faucial) tonsils lie in the lateral walls of the fauces.

3. The **laryngopharynx** (hypopharynx) extends from the hyoid bone to the oesophagus. It is inferior to the epiglottis and superior to the junction where the airway splits between the larynx and the esophagus. The lingual tonsils are found at the posterior base of the tongue which is near the opening of the oral cavity.

The Larynx

Inhaled air leaves the pharynx and enters the larynx, which is commonly known as the voice box as it houses the vocal folds that are responsible for sound production (phonation). It is found in the anterior neck, connecting the hypopharynx with the trachea, which extends vertically from the tip of the epiglottis to the inferior border of the cricoid cartilage (Fig. 7). At the top of the larynx is the epiglottis which acts as a flap that closes off the trachea during the act of swallowing to direct food into the oesophagus instead of the trachea. The larynx is a cartilaginous structure that surrounds and protects the glottis. The larynx begins at the level of vertebra C4 or C5 and ends at the level of vertebra C6. Essentially a cylinder, the larynx has incomplete cartilaginous walls that are stabilized by ligaments and skeletal muscles. Three large single cartilages form the larynx (thyroid cartilage, cricoid cartilage, and the epiglottis) connected by membranes and ligaments. The single laryngeal cartilages are:

The thyroid cartilage (*Adam's apple*) is the largest laryngeal cartilage formed by the fusion of two cartilage plates. Consisting of hyaline cartilage, it forms most of the anterior and lateral walls of the larynx. It is shaped like a triangular shield and is usually larger in males than in females due to male sex hormones stimulating its growth during puberty.

The thyroid cartilage sits superior to the cricoid cartilage, another hyaline cartilage. The posterior portion of the cricoid is greatly expanded, providing support in the absence of the thyroid cartilage, these two cartilages protect the glottis and the entrance to the trachea and their broad surface provide sites for the attachment of important laryngeal muscles and ligaments.

The epiglottis cartilage is a leaf-shaped piece of elastic cartilage located at the top of the larynx. It is inferiorly anchored at one end between the back of the tongue and the anterior rim of the thyroid cartilage. The free superior end bends up and down like a flap to open and close the opening into the larynx.

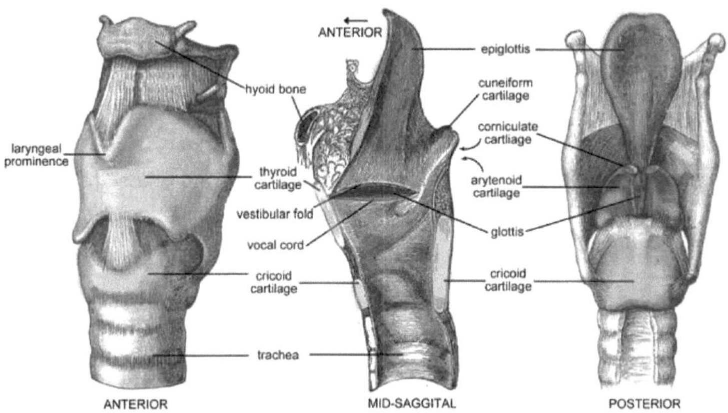

Fig. 7 Anterior, mid-sagittal (cut-away) and posterior views of the larynx

The larynx also contains three pairs of smaller hyaline cartilages. The arytenoid cartilages are located at the back of the larynx and attached to the cricoarytenoid muscles, anchored by the cricoid cartilage and attached to the vocal cords. They are the most important because they influence the position and tension of the vocal folds.

The corniculate cartilages are small and cone-shaped hyaline cartilages that sit on top of each of the arytenoid cartilages. During swallowing of food, the epiglottis bends down and meets the corniculate cartilages to close off the pathway to the trachea. In addition, the corniculate cartilages articulate with the arytenoid cartilages and they are involved with the opening and closing of the glottis and the production of sound.

The cuneiform cartilages are small elongated rod-like elastic cartilages located at the apex of each arytenoid cartilage, and at the base of the epiglottis above and anterior to the corniculate cartilage. In addition, it is lie within folds of tissue that extend between the lateral surface of each arytenoid cartilage and the epiglottis.

The various laryngeal cartilages are bound together by ligaments; additional ligaments attach the thyroid cartilage to the hyoid bone and the cricoid cartilage to the trachea. The vestibular ligaments and the vocal ligaments extend between the thyroid cartilage and the arytenoid cartilages.

The vestibular and vocal ligaments are covered by folds of laryngeal epithelium that project into glottis. The vestibular ligaments lie within the superior pair of folds, known as the vestibular folds. These folds, which relatively inelastic, help prevent foreign objects from entering the glottis and protect the more delicate vocal folds. The vestibular and vocal folds divide the larynx into (1) the vestibule (upper chamber), located above the vestibular folds; (2) the ventricle, the small middle chamber located between the vestibular and vocal folds; and (3) the infraglottic cavity, which extends from the vocal folds to the lower border of the cricoid cartilage (Fig. 8). The vocal cords, are flat triangular bands and white in colour because of their lack of blood supply (avascular) nature.

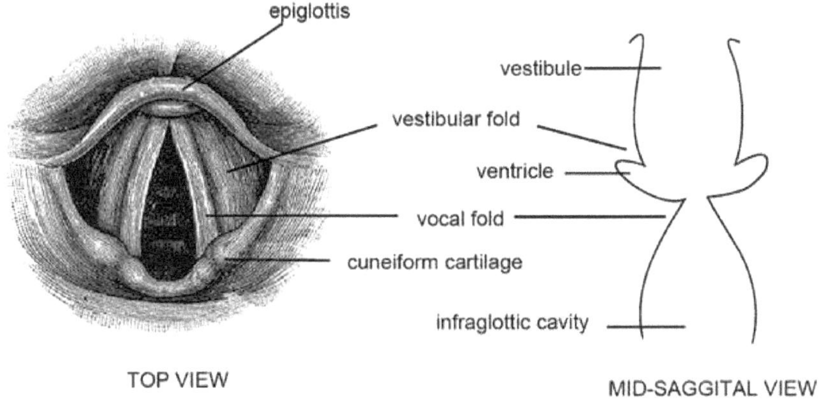

Fig. 8 Larynx opening at the glottis, showing the vocal and vestibular folds that separate the region into sub-cavities.

The Trachea

The epithelium of the larynx is continuous with that of the trachea, a tough, flexible tube with a diameter of about 2.5 cm and a length of about 11 cm. The trachea (windpipe) is a hollow tube connecting from the cricoid cartilage in the larynx to the primary bronchi of the lungs where it branches to form the right and left primary bronchi. There are 16–20 tracheal rings, which hold and support the trachea preventing it from collapsing in on itself but also provides some flexibility for any neck movement. Further downstream, along subsequent bronchi, the cartilage support becomes progressively smaller and less complete.

The mucosa of the trachea consists of pseudo stratified, ciliated columnar epithelium, while its submucosa contains cartilage, smooth muscle, and seromucous glands. The trachea divides into the main bronchi (primary bronchi) at the carina, with the right bronchus wider, shorter and more vertical than the left bronchus. This leads to increased chances of inhaled foreign particles depositing within the right bronchus. The right main bronchus bifurcates posterior and inferiorly into the right upper lobe bronchus and an intermediate bronchus. This bifurcation occurs earlier on the right than on the left lung in all models. The left bronchus passes inferolaterally at a greater angle from the vertical axis than the right bronchus. It is located anterior to the oesophagus and thoracic aorta and inferior to the aortic arch. Each main bronchi leads into the lung on its respective side (Fig. 9). The right main bronchus subdivides into three lobar (secondary) bronchi (right upper lobe bronchus, right middle lobe bronchus, and right lower lobe bronchus) while the left main bronchus divides into two (left upper lobe bronchus and left lower lobe bronchus). Each lobar bronchus serves as the airway to a specific lobe of the lung.

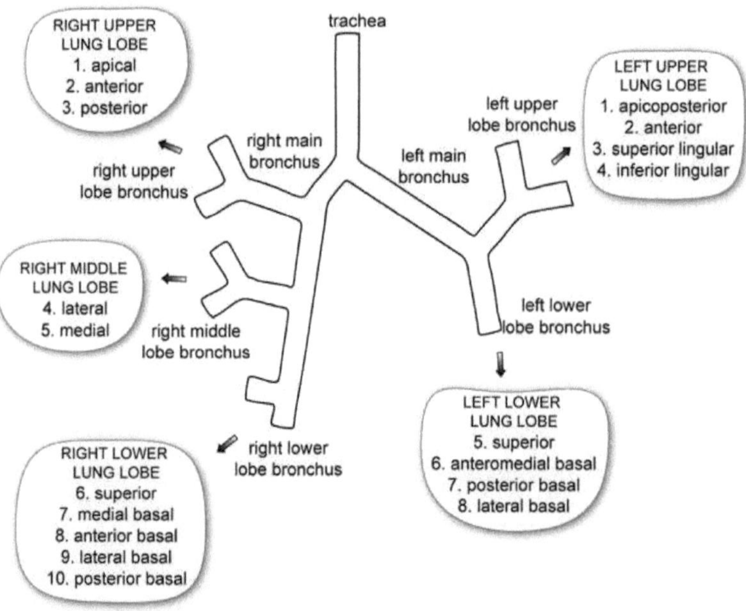

Fig. 9 Trachea branches

The Lungs

The left and right lungs are in the left and right pleural cavities, respectively. Each lung is a blunt cone, the tip, or apex, of which points superiorly. The apex on each side extends into the base of the neck superior to the first rib. The broad concave inferior portion, or base, of each lung rests on the superior surface of the diaphragm.

The lungs have distinct lobes that are separated by deep fissures. The right lung has three lobes; superior, middle, and inferior, separated by the horizontal and oblique fissures. The left lung has only two lobes; superior and inferior, separated by the oblique fissures. The right lung is broader than the left because most of the heart and great vessels project into the left thoracic cavity. However, the left lung is longer than the right lung because the diaphragm rises on the right side to accommodate the mass of the liver.

The curving anterior and lateral surfaces of each lung follow the inner contours of the rib cage. The medial surface, which contains the hilus, has a more irregular shape. The medial surfaces of both lungs bear grooves that mark the positions of the great vessels and the heart. The heart is located to the left of the midline, and the corresponding impression is larger in the left lung than in the right. In anterior view, the medial edge of the right lung forms a vertical line, whereas the medial margin of the left lung is indented at the cardiac notch.

Histology of Respiratory System

Conducting Airways

The airways of the lung provide a pathway for bringing external air to the gas exchange surfaces of the lung. They are organized in a tree-like configuration of rapidly branching tubes with progressively smaller diameters. Because these airways do not contain any gas exchange surfaces they are known as "conducting airways". The term "conducting" is also used because the movement of gas through these areas occurs by bulk flow, similar to air being blown through a straw.

The conducting airways of the lower respiratory tract begin with the trachea which divides into the two main bronchi that serve the right and left lungs, respectively. These in turn split into the lobar bronchi, each of which supplies an entire lobe of the lung. The lobar bronchi then progressively split into shorter and narrower airways until the final, smallest conducting airway known as the terminal bronchiole is reached. On average there are roughly 17 branch points between the trachea and any particular terminal bronchiole.

The histological architecture of all the conducting airways is roughly the same, and is organized as a series of concentric layers. All conducting airways are lined by the respiratory epithelium composed of a layer of respiratory epithelial cells which begin as a ciliated pseudostratified columnar epithelium in the trachea and slowly transition to that of a non-ciliated simple cuboidal epithelium in the terminal bronchioles. Mucin-secreting Goblet Cells are scattered throughout the respiratory epithelium with the greatest density in the trachea. Their density decreases as the airways progressively branch, completely disappearing by the terminal bronchioles.

The basic morphology of the conducting airways is similar and consists of a surface epithelium composed largely of ciliated and secretory cells overlying subepithelial tissue that consists predominantly of connective tissues and glands (Fig 10). The proportion and type of these elements vary at different levels of the conducting system.

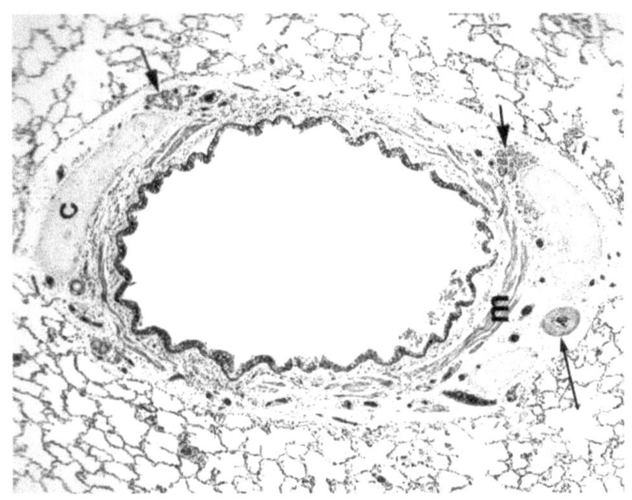

Fig 10 Conducting airway (hematoxylin-eosin stain). Subsegmental bronchus showing cartilage (c), mucous glands (*shortarrows*), bronchial artery (*long arrow*), and muscle (m).

Respiratory Epithelium:

The tracheal and proximal bronchial epithelium are composed predominantly of tall, columnar ciliated and goblet cells, and smaller, somewhat triangular, basal cells (Fig 11). Ciliated cells are about five times more numerous than goblet cells in the central airways, and the ratio is even greater peripherally. They have thin, tapering bases that are attached firmly to the underlying basal lamina. The cells are also attached to one another at their apical surfaces by tight junctions, forming a barrier physically impermeable to most substances, and laterally to one another and to basal cells by desmosomes. Intercellular spaces containing numerous microvilli are present between the cells, especially at their basal aspects. Emanating from the surface of each ciliated cell are approximately 200 to 250 cilia, as well as numerous shorter microvilli (Fig 12), which, in addition to microvilli located in the intercellular space, are important in the transepithelial movement of fluid and electrolytes.

21

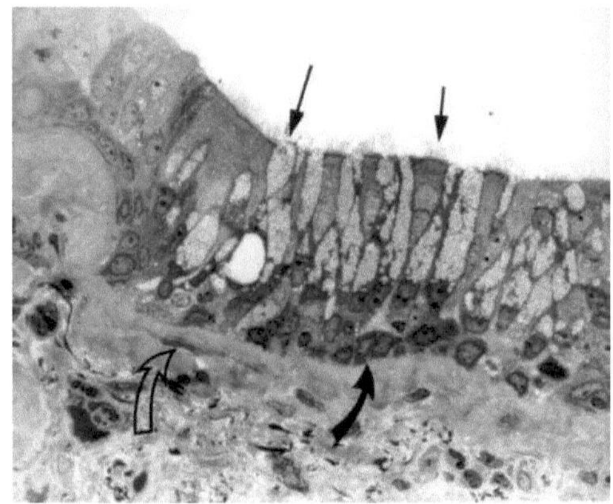

Fig 11 Conducting airway epithelium and lamina propria (electron micrograph). Ciliated cell (short straight arrow), goblet cell (long straight arrow), basal cell (black curved arrow), and subepithelial fibroblast (empty curved arrow).

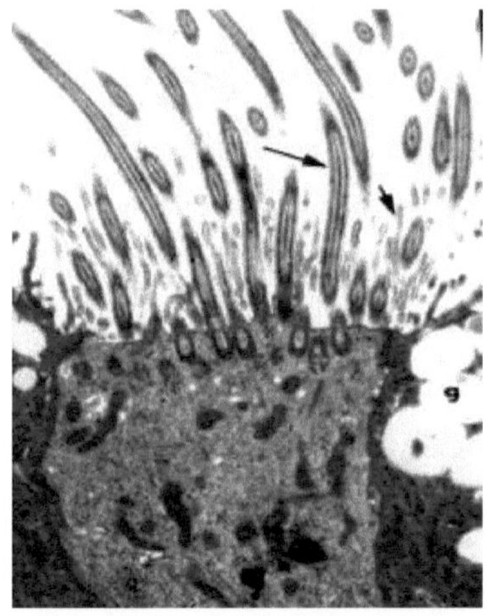

Fig 12 Ciliated cell (electron micrograph). Apical portion of cell showing cilia (*long arrow*) and microvilli (*short arrow*). Secretory granules (g) of a goblet cell can be seen in the adjacent cell.

Goblet cells are modified simple columnar epithelial cells, having a height of four times that of their width. The cytoplasm of goblet cells tends to be displaced toward the basal end of the cell body by the large mucin granules, which accumulate near the apical surface of the cell along the Golgi apparatus, which lies between the granules and the nucleus. This gives the basal part of the cell a basophilic staining because of nucleic acids within the nucleus and rough endoplasmic reticulum staining with hematoxylin. Mucin within the granules stains pale in routine histology sections, primarily because these carbohydrate-rich proteins are washed out in the preparation of microscopy samples. However, they stain easily with the PAS staining method, which colours them magenta.

Goblet cells are found scattered among the epithelial lining of organs, such as the intestinal and respiratory tracts. They are found inside the trachea, bronchi, and larger bronchioles in the respiratory tract, small intestines, the large intestine, and conjunctiva in the upper eyelid. Goblet cells are a source of mucus in tears and secrete different types of mucins onto the ocular surface, especially in the conjunctiva. In the lacrimal glands, mucus is synthetized by acinar cells instead.

The main role of goblet cells is to secrete mucus in order to protect the mucous membranes where they are found. Goblet cells accomplish this by secreting mucins, large glycoproteins formed mostly by carbohydrates. The gel-like properties of mucins are given by its glycans (bound carbohydrates) attracting relatively large quantities of water. On the inner surface of the human intestine, it forms a 200 μm thick layer (less in other animals) that lubricates and protects the wall of the organ. Distinct forms of mucin are produced in different organs: while MUC2 is prevalent in the intestine, MUC5AC and MUC5B are the main forms found in the human airway. Mucins are stored in granules inside the goblet cells before being released to the lumen of the organ. Secretion may be stimulated by irritants such as dust and smoke, especially in the airway. Other stimuli are microbes such as viruses and bacteria.

Basal cells are relatively small, somewhat triangular cells whose bases are attached to the basement membrane and whose apices normally do not reach the airway lumen. They are more abundant in the proximal airways, where they form a more or less continuous layer, and gradually diminish in number distally, so that they are difficult to identify in bronchioles. They function as a reserve from which the epithelium is repopulated, both normally and after airway injury, and are involved in the attachment of columnar epithelial cells to the basement membrane.

Clara cells are a cuboidal epithelial cell found in the lining of the terminal and the respiratory bronchioles of the lungs. They are nonciliated, and secrete surfactant, like the type II alveolar epithelial cells found deeper in the bronchial tree. These cells, along with goblet cells, provide secretions for the respiratory tract. The secretion is a mucus-poor protein that coats the epithelium. However, one of the main functions of Clara cells is to protect the bronchiolar epithelium. They do this by secreting a small variety of products, including Clara cell secretory protein (CCSP) and a solution similar to the component of the lung surfactant. They are also responsible for detoxifying harmful substances inhaled into the lungs. Clara cells accomplish this with cytochrome P450 enzymes found in their smooth endoplasmic reticulum. Clara cells also multiply and differentiate into ciliated cells (most notably the type II pneumocytes) to regenerate the bronchiolar epithelium.

Neuroendocrine cells are cells that receive neuronal input (neurotransmitters released by nerve cells or neurosecretory cells) and, as a consequence of this input, release message molecules (hormones) to the blood. In this way they bring about an integration between the nervous system and the endocrine system, a process known as neuroendocrine integration. An example of a neuroendocrine cell is a cell of the adrenal medulla (innermost part of the adrenal gland), which releases adrenaline to the blood. The adrenal medullary cells are controlled by the sympathetic division of the autonomic nervous system. These cells are modified postganglionic neurons. Autonomic nerve fibers lead directly to them from the central nervous system. The adrenal medullary hormones are kept in vesicles much in the same way neurotransmitters are kept in neuronal vesicles. Hormonal effects can last up to ten times longer than those of neurotransmitters[citation needed]. Sympathetic nerve fiber impulses stimulate the release of adrenal medullary hormones. In this way the sympathetic division of the autonomic nervous system and the medullary secretions function together.

Pulmonary neuroendocrine cells (PNEC) are specialized airway epithelial cells that occur as solitary cells or as clusters called neuroepithelial bodies (NEB) in the lung, (fig 13). They are located in the nasal respiratory epithelium, laryngeal mucosa and throughout the entire respiratory tract from the trachea to the terminal airways. PNEC and NEB exist from fetal stage and neonatal stage in lungs airway area. These cells are bottle- or flask-like in shape, and reach from the basement membrane to the lumen. They can be distinguished by their profile of bioactive amines and peptides, namely serotonin, calcitonin, calcitonin gene-related peptide (CGRP), chromogranin A, gastrin-releasing peptide (GRP), and cholecystokinin.

The major center of neuroendocrine integration in the body is found in the hypothalamus and the pituitary gland. Here hypothalamic neurosecretory cells release factors to the blood. Some of these factors (releasing hormones), released at the hypothalamic median eminence, control the secretion of pituitary hormones, while others (the hormones oxytocin and vasopressin) are released directly into the blood. However, the main function of neuroendocrine cells is hypoxia detection.

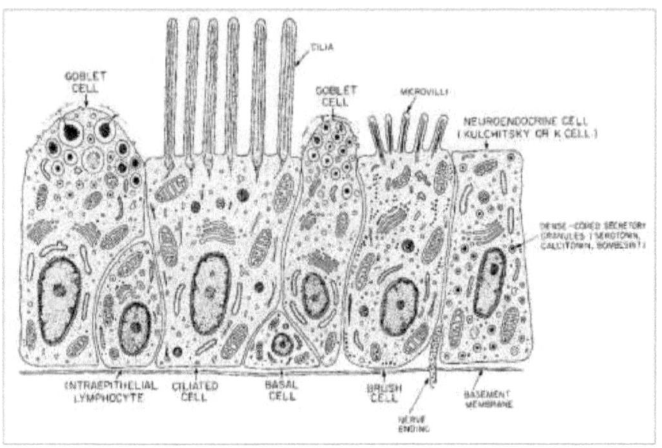

Fig 13 shows neuroendocrine cells

Cells of the immune system are present within the epithelium of all conducting airways. Dendritic and Langerhans' cells are structurally similar cells that possess elongated cytoplasmic extensions and an organelle-rich cytoplasm; Langerhans' cells have characteristic pentalaminar cytoplasmic structures termed Birbeck granules.

Dendritic cells are found throughout the lung, including the alveolar septa, peribronchiolar connective tissue, and bronchus-associated lymphoid tissue; Langerhans' cells appear to be present only within airway epithelium. In this location, their number is considerably greater in proximal than in distal branches. Langerhans' cells express cell surface receptors for immunoglobulins, and it is believed that they act as antigen-processing and antigen-presenting cells and as stimulators of T-cell proliferation.

Lymphocytes (predominantly T cells) are present throughout the conducting airway epithelium, usually singly. Though they are undoubtedly involved in processing and reacting to inhaled antigens, it is also possible that they have a role in modifying airway epithelial cell function. Greater numbers of lymphocytes can be seen as lymphoid aggregates in the lamina propria and submucosa (bronchusassociated lymphoid tissue), usually in the setting of acute or chronic airway injury.

Mast cells are also found in small numbers within the airway epithelium. A basement membrane underlies the epithelium over its entire basal aspect. Its primary function is to provide an attachment for the epithelium to the underlying connective tissue. On the epithelial side, this attachment is mediated by adhesion molecules and by hemidesmosomal junctions with basal cells; on the opposite side, anchoring fibrils emanate from the basement membrane and intertwine with collagen fibers in the upper lamina propria.

Submucosa and Lamina Propria

Submucosa

The subepithelial tissue can be subdivided into a lamina propria, situated between the basement membrane and the muscularis mucosa, and a submucosa, consisting of all the remaining airway tissue. The submucosa contains cartilage, muscle, and other supportive connective tissue elements, as well as the major portion of the tracheobronchial glands. The submucosa is the layer of dense irregular connective tissue or loose connective tissue that supports the mucosa, as well as joins the mucosa to the bulk of overlying smooth muscle (fibers running circularly within layer of longitudinal muscle).

The respiratory mucosa is made up of the epithelium and supporting lamina propria). The epithelium is tall columnar pseudostratified with cilia and goblet cells. The supporting lamina propria underneath the epithelium contains elastin, that plays a role in the elastic recoil of the trachea during inspiration and expiration, together with blood vessels that warm the air.

The sub-mucosa contains glands which are mixed sero-mucous glands, (fig 14). The watery secretions from the serous glands humidify the inspired air. The mucous, together with mucous from the goblet cells traps particles from the air which are transported upwards towards the pharynx by the cilia on the epithlium. This helps to keep the lungs free of particles and bacteria.

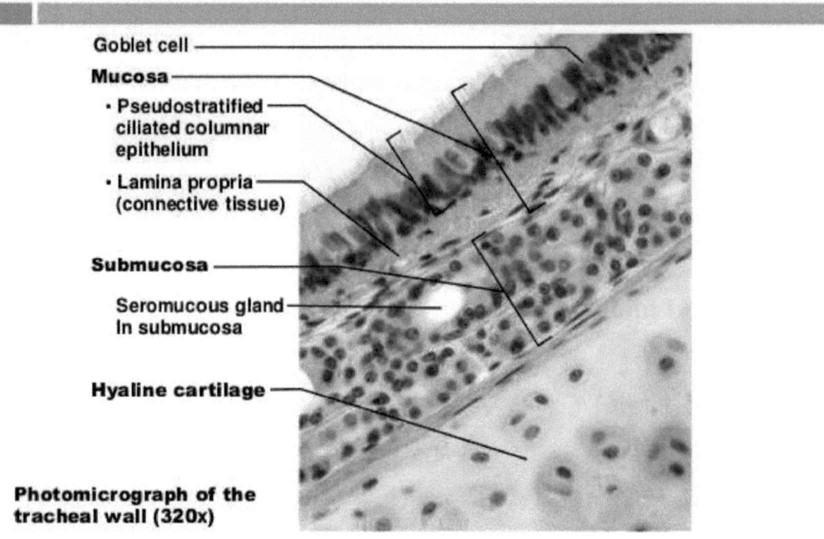

Fig 14 shows submucosa and seromucous gland

Lamina Propria

The lamina propria is a constituent of the moist linings known as mucous membranes or mucosa, which line various tubes in the body (such as the respiratory tract, the gastrointestinal tract, and the urogenital tract). The lamina propria (more correctly lamina propria mucosæ) is a thin layer of loose connective tissue, or dense irregular connective tissue, which lies beneath the epithelium and together with the epithelium constitutes the mucosa. As its Latin name indicates it is a characteristic component of the mucosa, "the mucosa's own special layer". Thus the term mucosa or mucous membrane always refers to the combination of the epithelium plus the lamina propria.

28

The connective tissue of the lamina propria is very loose allowing it to be very cell rich. The cell population of the lamina propria is very varied including, for example, fibroblasts, lymphocytes, plasma cells, macrophages, eosinophilic leukocytes, and mast cells.[2] It provides support and nutrition to the epithelium, as well as the means to bind to the underlying tissue. Irregularities in the connective tissue surface, such as papillae found in the tongue, increase the area of contact of the lamina propria and the epithelium. The lamina propria contains capillaries and a central lacteal (lymph vessel) in the small intestine, as well as lymphoid tissue. Lamina propria also contains glands with the ducts opening on to the mucosal epithelium, that secrete mucus and serous secretions. The lamina propria is also rich in immune cells known as lymphocytes. A majority of these cells are IgA-secreting B cells.

The lamina propria is a loose connective tissue, hence it is not as fibrous as the underlying connective tissue of the submucosa. The connective tissue and architecture of the lamina propria is very compressible and elastic, this can be seen in organs that require expansion such as the bladder. The collagen in the lamina propria of elastic organs has been shown to play a major role in mechanical function. In the bladder the collagen composition of its lamina propria allows for structure, tensile strength, and compliance, through complex coiling. It has been suggested that myofibroblasts also reside in the lamina propria of several organs. These cells have characteristics of both smooth muscle and fibroblasts.

The lamina propria may also be rich in vascular networks, lymphatic vessels, elastic fibers, and smooth muscle fascicles from the muscularis mucosae. Afferent and efferent nerve endings can be found in the lamina propria as well. Immune cells as well as lymphoid tissue, including lymphoid nodules and capillaries, may be present. Smooth muscle fibers may be in the lamina propria of some tissues, such as the intestinal villi. It is practically void of fat cells. Lymphatics penetrate the mucosa and lie below the basement membrane of the epithelium, from there they drain the lamina propria. The fast rate of cell death and regeneration of the epithelium leaves behind many apoptotic cell bodies. This have been found to go into the lamina propria, most of which are inside its macrophages.

Respiratory Tissue

There are three major cell types in the alveolar wall. Type I pneumocyte cells (also called type I alveolar cells or squamous alveolar cells) are extremely attenuated cells that line the alveolar surfaces of the lungs. They cover 95% of the alveolar surface, with type II pneumocytes covering the remainder. These cells are so thin (sometimes only 25 nm) that the electron microscope was needed to prove that all alveoli are covered with an epithelial lining. It is important that these cells are thin so that gas exchange between the alveoli and blood can occur easily. Their main role is to provide a barrier of minimal thickness that is readily permeable to gases such as oxygen and carbon dioxide. Organelles of Type 1 pneumocyte cells such as the endoplasmic reticulum, Golgi apparatus and mitochondria are clustered around the nucleus. This leaves large areas of cytoplasm virtually free of organelles and reduces the thickness of the cell, thus reducing the thickness of the blood-air barrier. The cytoplasm in the thin portion contains pinocytotic vesicles, which may play a role in the turnover of surfactant and the removal of small particulate contaminants from the outer surface. (However, type 2 pneumocytes are primarily responsible for secretion of surfactant). In addition to desmosomes, all type I pneumocyte cells have occluding junctions that prevent the leakage of tissue fluid into the alveolar air space.

Type I pneumocytes are unable to replicate and are susceptible to toxic insults. In the event of damage, Type II cells can proliferate and/or differentiate into type I cells to compensate.

Type II (Great Alveolar) cells that secrete pulmonary surfactant to lower the surface tension of water and allows the membrane to separate, therefore increasing its capability to exchange gases. Surfactant is continuously released by exocytosis. It forms an underlying aqueous protein-containing hypophase and an overlying phospholipid film composed primarily of dipalmitoyl phosphatidylcholine.

Type II pneumocytes also called alveolar type II cells, great alveolar cells or septal cells are granular and roughly cuboidal in shape. Type II pneumocytes are typically found at the alveolar-septal junction. Although they only comprise <5% of the alveolar surface, they are relatively numerous (60% of alveolar epithelial cells). Type II tend to be located near corners where alveoli meet. Their cytoplasm contains a welldeveloped endoplasmic reticulum, a prominent Golgi complex, and numerous membrane-bound, secretory granules (Fig 15). The latter contain characteristic lamellar inclusions that are the source of surfactant, the substance responsible for modifying alveolar surface tension. Type II cells have a number of other important functions. A small number are mitotically active and are able to differentiate into type I cells, repopulating the alveolar surface as the latter die. There is also evidence that type II cells synthesize a variety of substances involved in alveolar structure and defense, including fibronectin and _1-antitrypsin, and are able to suppress lymphocyte proliferation and enhance macrophage function in the alveolar septa. Surfactant can be identified on transmission electron microscopy as an extremely thin (4 nm) layer of osmiophilic material that covers the alveolar epithelial surface. It appears to consist of two components: (1) a film facing the alveolar airspace, which is composed of densely spaced, highly surface-active phospholipids, and (2) a deep layer containing surface-active phospholipids in a different physicochemical configuration and linked to proteins. Components of the superficial layer are thought to be recruited from the deeper layer (hypophase) during expansion of the lung and may reenter it at low lung volumes. The hypophase contains aggregates of lipid termed tubular myelin that have a characteristic fingerprint-like pattern.

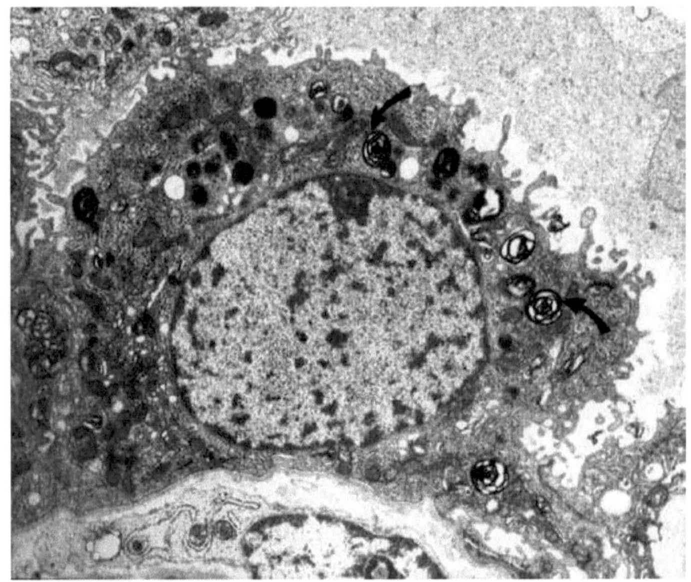

Fig 15 Type II epithelial cell (electron micrograph). Secretory granules with lamellar inclusions (arrows).

An alveolar macrophage (or dust cell) is a type of macrophage found in the pulmonary alveolus (Fig 16), near the pneumocytes, but separated from the wall. Activity of the alveolar macrophage is relatively high, because they are located at one of the major boundaries between the body and the outside world. Dust cells are another name for monocyte derivatives in the lungs that reside on respiratory surfaces and clean off particles such as dust or microorganisms. Alveolar macrophages are frequently seen to contain granules of exogenous material such as particulate carbon that they have picked up from respiratory surfaces. Such black granules may be especially common in smoker's lungs or long-term city dwellers.

Inhaled air may contain particles or organisms which would be pathogenic. The respiratory pathway is a prime site for exposure to pathogens and toxic substances.

The respiratory tree, comprising the larynx, trachea, and bronchioles, is lined by ciliated epithelia cells that are continually exposed to harmful matter. When these offensive agents infiltrate the superficial barriers, the body's immune system responds in an orchestrated defense involving a litany of specialized cells which target the threat, neutralize it, and clean up the remnants of the battle.

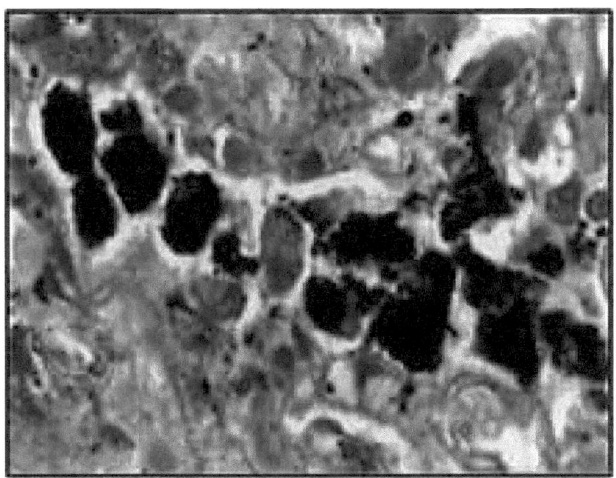

Fig 16 Micrograph of carbon-laden macrophages in the lung, H&E stain

Alveolar macrophages are phagocytes that play a critical role in homeostasis, host defense, the response to foreign substances, and tissue remodeling. Since alveolar macrophages are pivotal regulators of local immunological homeostasis, their population density is decisive for the many processes of immunity in the lungs. They are highly adaptive components of the innate immune system and can be specifically modified to whatever functions needed depending on their state of differentiation and micro-environmental factors encountered. Alveolar macrophages release numerous secretory products and interact with other cells and molecules through the expression of several surface receptors. Alveolar macrophages are also involved in the phagocytosis of apoptotic and necrotic cells that have undergone cell-death. They must be selective of the material that is phagocytized because normal cells and structures of the body must not be compromised. To combat infection, the phagocytes of the innate immune system facilitates many pattern recognition receptors (PRR) to help recognize pathogen-associated molecular patterns (PAMPs) on the surface of pathogenic microorganisms. PAMPs all have the common features of being unique to a group of pathogens but invariant in their basic structure; and are essential for pathogenicity (ability of an organism to produce an infectious disease in another organism).

Pulmonary Vasculature

Pulmonary Arteries

Most individuals have two to four bronchial arteries, a relatively common pattern being one on the right (originating from the third intercostal artery) and two on the left (arising directly from the aorta). At the hila, the vessels form an intercommunicating circular arc around the main bronchi from which several branches (usually two or three on opposite sides of the airway wall) extend into the peribronchial connective tissue (Figure 10). These branches send smaller twigs into the bronchial wall that ramify to form a vascular plexus in the submucosa. The latter can comprise as much as 10 to 20% of the volume of the normal subepithelial tissue, and it has been hypothesized that significant airway narrowing may occur when these vessels become congested. Most arteries stop at the level of the terminal bronchioles. The bronchial circulation has a dual venous drainage. One portion, related to the trachea and proximal bronchi, drains into the bronchial veins to the right side of the heart via the azygos and hemiazygos veins. The other, which drains the major portion of the intrapulmonary bronchial flow, originates in anastomoses with small precapillary and postcapillary pulmonary vessels and courses via the pulmonary veins into the left atrium.

Pulmonary Veins

Unlike pulmonary arteries, pulmonary veins and venules are not associated with airways and course instead in the parenchyma or in the connective tissue septa that delimit the secondary lobules. As in the pulmonary arterial system, numerous supernumerary vessels join the veins as they run to the hilum. Histologically, pulmonary venules are indistinguishable from arterioles. Veins have a variable number of elastic laminae, between which are small bundles of smooth muscle cells. No valves are present within venous lumina. However, regularly spaced annular constrictions related to local accumulations of smooth muscle have been identified in the veins of some animals and have been hypothesized to be important in the control of pulmonary blood flow.

Chapter Two

Physiological of Respiratory System

Physiology of the Nose and Nasal Cavity

The physiology of airflow through the nose is not complicated. Inspired air flows uniformly over the nasal turbinates, which add heat and moisture to the air. By the time the air reaches our lungs it is warmed and humidified supporting comfortable breathing. The nose is nature's humidifier. When we are congested (such as with a cold) and we breathe through our mouth at night we awake with a sore dry throat. The nose is not necessary for breathing, just to do so comfortably. When the septum is perforated the normal pattern of airflow through the nose is disrupted. Inspired air beings to recirculate, swirling through the nose, much like calm flowing water turning to rapids in a stream.

The recirculation of inspired air "steals" more than its fair share of moisture and heat on its way back out of the nose through the perforation causing excessive drying of the delicate nasal mucosa. Alternately inspired air may simply become trapped in the perforation like a whirlpool. This abnormal airflow through the nose leads to excessive drying of the mucosal membrane. The septal perforation itself becomes crusted, bloody, and occasionally infected with bacteria that easily penetrate the damaged mucosa and cartilage. Patients often present to their physician with blocked nasal passages from excessive crusts, foul smelling pus in the nose, and nosebleeds. If the septal perforation is left untreated the crust, infection, and bleeding damage more cartilage and the septal perforation slowly becomes larger destabilizing the nose leading to potential collapse and worsening symptoms.

Physiology of the Pharynx:

The pharynx assists to provide a pathway for both the respiratory system and digestive system since air and food pass through it, the air or food is directed down the correct pathway, either the trachea or the oesophagus, by being controlled by the epiglottis. The epiglottis is a flap of elastic cartilage tissue that acts as a lid to cover the trachea when food is swallowed in order to prevent objects entering the larynx. During swallowing, the soft palate and its uvula point upwards closing the nasopharynx so that neither air nor food can pass through it, thus breathing is momentarily stopped. The connection opens and closes to equalize the air pressure in the middle ear to that of the atmosphere for the conduction of sound. The surface of the nasopharynx is covered by pseudo-stratified columnar epithelium.

This is the same epithelium found in the nasal cavity and similarly the same mechanism of mucous secretion from goblet cells in the epithelium to filter, warm, and humidify the inhaled air occurs here. In the oropharynx and laryngopharynx, the surface is lined with non-keratinizing stratified squamous epithelium which is needed as it is exposed to food moving through the passageway.

Physiology of the Larynx

The ciliated mucous lining of the larynx further contributes towards the respiratory system's ability to remove foreign particles and to warm and humidify the inhaled air (the same physiological feature as the nasal cavity). During intentional swallowing the back of the tongue that is joined to the top of the larynx, pushes upwards, forcing the epiglottis to close over the glottis, preventing food or foreign objects to enter the larynx. If the items do enter the larynx and contact the vocal folds, stimulation of the larynx muscles causes a cough reflex to try and expel the items in order to prevent choking. The other important function of the larynx is sound generation (phonation), where the pitch and volume of sounds are manipulated by the body.

Sounds generated at the larynx are caused by the expired air released from the lungs that pass through the glottis and hence the vocal cords. By flexing and reflexing muscles in the larynx, the arytenoid cartilages are forced to pivot at its base (i.e. at the cricoid cartilage) to bring together or separate the vocal cords for speech or breathing respectively. The vocal and cricothyroid muscles then control their length and tension.

This variable tension in the vocal cords allows a wide range of pitch and tones to be produced. Generally the tenser the vocal cords, the faster they vibrate and the higher the pitch. As young boy's experience puberty, the larynx enlarges which produces thicker and longer vocal cords. This leads to the cords, vibrating more slowly and his voice becomes deeper. Louder sounds can be achieved through

greater exhalation force from the diaphragm, creating stronger vibrations of the vocal cords. Just like guitar strings the vocal cords produce a vibrating buzzing sound and the final sound produced is dependent on the surrounding resonating chambers of the pharynx, mouth, and nose and also the geometry of the tongue and lips.

Physiology of the Tracheobronchial Tree and Lung Airways

The tracheobronchial tree conducts the inspired air to and from the alveoli. During inhalation the distal end and bifurcation of the trachea are displaced downwards, which is important for facilitating inspiration. The epithelial changes in the bronchi reflect the physiological functions of the airway. For example the ciliated columnar epithelium in the early branch generations allow for both heating and conditioning of the air as well as filtering through mucociliary action to remove mucous secretions in an upward motion towards the oesophagus. In the distal branches, the epithelium becomes cuboidal to allow for gas exchange. The cartilage support around the trachea and early branches also changes, progressively diminishing in order to maintain patency of the smaller airways. During gas exchange oxygen is brought into the body and is exchanged with carbon dioxide that is produced from cell metabolism. This occurs in the alveolar-capillary network which consists of a dense mesh-like network of the respiratory bronchioles, the alveolar ducts, the alveoli, and the pulmonary capillary bed. At the gas exchange surface of the alveoli is a lining that is $1–2$ μm thick where O2 and CO2 passively diffuse across and into plasma and red blood cells. The diffusion occurs between the alveolar gas and blood in the pulmonary capillaries within less than one second.

Chapter Three

Chronic Obstructive Pulmonary Disease (COPD)

Chronic obstructive pulmonary disease (COPD) is the fifth cause of morbidity and mortality in the developed world and represents a substantial economic and social burden. Patients experience a progressive deterioration up to end-stage COPD, characterised by very severe airflow limitation, severely limited and declining performance status with chronic respiratory failure, advanced age, multiple comorbidities and severe systemic manifestations/complications.

COPD is an umbrella term encompassing two distinct pathological processes: *chronic bronchitis* which clinically manifests itself as a chronic productive cough and *pulmonary emphysema* characterized by destruction and enlargement of pulmonary alveoli.

Two of the world's leading respiratory disease bodies, the American Thoracic Society (ATS), and the European Respiratory Society (ERS), have defined COPD as "*a preventable and treatable disease state characterised by airflow limitation that is not fully reversible. The airflow limitation is usually progressive and associated with an abnormal inflammatory response of the lungs to noxious particles or gases, primarily caused by cigarette smoking. Although COPD affects the lungs, it also produces significant systemic consequences*".

This is in accord with the 2009 Global Initiative for Chronic Obstructive Lung Disease (GOLD) which states that COPD is "a *preventable and treatable disease with some significant extra-pulmonary effects that may contribute to the severity in individual patients. Its pulmonary component is characterized by airflow limitation that is not fully reversible. The airflow limitation is usually progressive and associated with an abnormal inflammatory response of the lung to noxious particles or gases.*".

In the classical view of the disease, COPD was considered a respiratory disease only, based on the presence of chronic airflow limitation. In the last decades however, important manifestations beyond the lungs were described. These extra-pulmonary manifestations are also referred to as the systemic effects of COPD and are included in the most recent GOLD definition of the disease. These effects include weight loss and nutritional abnormalities, skeletal muscle dysfunction, increased risk of cardiovascular disease, hormonal and metabolic disturbances, osteoporosis and anxiety and depression. The new understanding of COPD has important clinical implications. In addition to traditional pharmacological therapy focused on treating chronic airflow limitation, management of COPD now requires a more holistic approach. Pulmonary rehabilitation programs aimed at reversing some of the extra-pulmonary manifestations of advanced COPD have been developed.

Significant improvements in exercise tolerance, nutritional status and health-related quality of life were achieved by pulmonary rehabilitation and this type of non-pharmacological therapy is now considered one of the essential components of disease management. While the list of systemic effects of COPD is still growing, the drivers of these manifestations are only partially understood. Systemic inflammation is recognized as one of the key mechanisms behind many of the extra-pulmonary manifestations. In addition to an amplified inflammatory response of the respiratory tract to cigarette smoke and other irritants, a low-grade persistent abnormal inflammatory response is present in the systemic circulation of patients with COPD. This reaction is characterized by enhanced numbers of leukocytes in the circulation and increased circulating concentrations of acute-phase proteins, such as C-reactive protein (CRP) and fibrinogen along with acute-phase cytokines like tumour necrosis factor-α (TNF-α) and interleukin-6 (IL-6).

The origin of this low-grade systemic inflammation is unclear, although there are several possible mechanisms. The lack of correlation between inflammatory markers in respiratory samples and values in blood in COPD patients, suggests that the systemic inflammatory response is not a result of "spilling over" of pulmonary inflammation into the systemic compartment. There is evidence showing that cigarette smoking itself can cause systemic inflammation, which persists long after quitting. Also, other organs may contribute to continuous systemic inflammation in COPD. Increased plasma TNF-α levels were observed after submaximal exercise in patients with severe COPD, suggesting that exercising muscle is a possible site of origin. In addition, there's a growing scientific interest in bone marrow and fat mass as potential sources of pro-inflammatory mediators in COPD. Although it has recently been suggested that COPD should be considered a "chronic systemic inflammatory syndrome", there are several other potential mechanisms contributing to the systemic manifestations of the disease. These include semi-starvation, deconditioning, aging and chronic gas exchange abnormalities.

Aetiology of COPD

The Role of Smoking

Tobacco smoking is the main aetiological factor for the development of COPD. Cigarette smoking is estimated in western societies to account for around 85% of the risk of developing COPD. Moreover, the progressive deterioration in airways obstruction as measured by the rate of decline in the forced expiratory volume in one second (FEV_1), relates directly to the amount of tobacco smoked and years that tobacco has been smoked. The risks of dyspnoea, cough, wheezing and mucous production are increased by active cigarette smoking and that these features are directly related to the amount of cigarettes smoked.

The aim of smoking cessation is to slow the rate of decline of ventilatory function, dyspnoea, and disability. After cessation of smoking, the progressive decline in lung and airway function returns to levels that are normally associated with ageing. Indeed, there is often a small improvement in airway obstruction within a year after cessation of smoking, compared with the accelerated rate of decline in those patients who continue to smoke. These changes in airway obstruction are illustrated in Figure (17). Nevertheless, despite extensive publicity campaigns in the media to raise awareness of the health risks associated with smoking, smokers with COPD and other respiratory complaints continue to find it difficult to stop smoking. In an attempt to deal with this issue, an ERS Task Force has issued guidelines to patients to help them stop smoking.

Smoking is a major cause of death worldwide which resulted in 4.83 million deaths in the world for the year 2000. COPD accounted for 0.97 million of these deaths, whereas cardiovascular disease and lung cancer were estimated to have caused 1.69 million and 0.85 million deaths respectively. The 2004 report by the United States Surgeon General has also noted *"a relationship between active smoking and COPD mortality and general mortality and morbidity"*. In addition, although individuals with COPD have more frequent acute chest illnesses than people without COPD, mortality from COPD and the rate of decline of lung function are not always associated with cough and mucus hypersecretion.

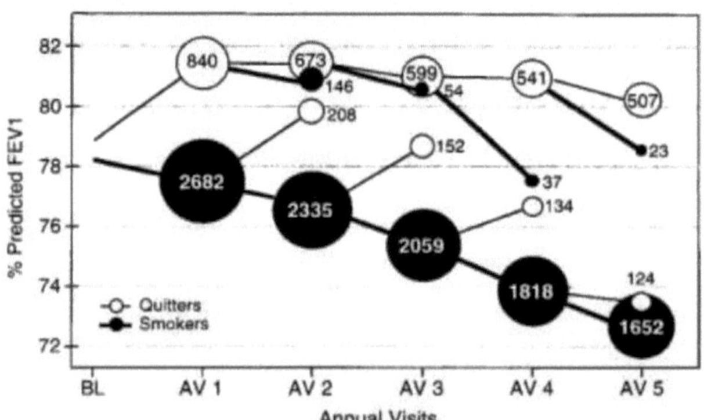

Fig 17. Lung function improved during Year 1 among quitters, but declined among continuing smokers. The subsequent rate of decline is twice as great among continuing smokers as among sustained quitters. Those who relapsed lost function and those who delayed quitting benefited regardless of when they quit.

There is mounting evidence that inhaling other peoples' tobacco smoke can have adverse health effects in those who do not smoke themselves. Although there is a paucity of relevant data in the literature, excess sputum production and breathlessness are believed to adversely affect people who passively inhale cigarette smoke. The U.S. Department of Health and Human Services (2004) considers that passive smoking in adult's results in increased rates of decline in lung function which is associated with dyspnoea and limitation of daily activities.

How Does Smoking Contribute to COPD?

The air you breathe travels down through the windpipe, eventually making its way into bronchial tubes. Bronchial tubes then stretch out into much smaller tubes known as bronchioles, which have minuscule clusters of air sacs at the end called alveoli.

Within the small air sacs are tiny blood vessels known as capillaries. When you inhale, the oxygen moves through the air sacs and into the blood of the capillaries that are located within the air sacs. Simultaneously, carbon dioxide is moved from the blood vessels into the air sacs in a process known as gas exchange.

The elasticity in the air sacs enables this exchange to occur smoothly as they inflate and deflate with each breath. People who smoke suffer lung damage which allows less air to flow in and out of the air pathways due to:

- Stiffening of air sacs
- Degradation of wall between air sacs
- Thickening and inflammation of air pathway walls
- Increasing mucus in the air pathways, causing build-up and air obstruction.

Cigarette smoke contains harmful toxins that affect lung functionality. Toxins that are inhaled directly into the lungs over prolonged periods of time can lead to high levels of abnormal lung irritation, causing the onset of COPD. As long-term exposure to cigarette smoke continues, the lungs incur more damage, including lung inflammation, and breakdown of the lung's filter system.

Can You Reverse Cigarette Damage?

Unfortunately, there is no cure for COPD. Damage to the lungs can't be reversed. COPD is treated using several different methods including changes in lifestyle, therapy, and prescription drugs. When used in combination, these treatment methods can slow down the progression of the disease and bring relief to the patient by causing symptoms to subside. The best way to stop the disease from worsening is for people who smoke to quit immediately and avoid secondhand smoke. People who continue to smoke put themselves at increased risk of accelerating the disease and its symptoms, as well as premature death.

Smoking Cessation and COPD

Smoking cessation is the single most effective—and cost-effective—treatment for COPD. Furthermore, smoking cessation is associated with a reduction in the risk of developing stroke, coronary heart disease, several types of cancer, and it is associated to an increased life expectancy. Despite the ongoing inflammatory process, there is increasing evidence that the rate of development of COPD can be reduced when patients at risk of developing the disease stop smoking.

The first indications came from longitudinal cohort studies which showed that subjects who continued to smoke had a much steeper decline in lung function than those who had stopped smoking. The Lung Health Study confirmed that smoking cessation could reduce this smoking-related precipitous decline in lung function. It was a randomized clinical trial designed to determine the potential benefits of smoking cessation. All participants had, as an inclusion criterion, asymptomatic airway obstruction. The special intervention participants received a smoking cessation program and were compared with usual care participants. Vital status was followed up to 14.5 years. The smoking intervention program consisted of a 10-week smoking cessation program that included a strong physician message and 12 group sessions using behavior modification and nicotine gum, plus either ipratropium or a placebo inhaler. At 5 years, 21.7% of special intervention participants had stopped smoking since study entry, compared with 5.4% of usual care participants. Smoking intervention participants had smaller declines in FEV-1 than usual care participants. Men who quit at the beginning of the study had an FEV-1 rate of decline of 30.2 mL/year, whereas women who quit declined at 21.5 mL/year. Men continuing to smoke throughout declined by 66.1 mL/year, and women continuing to smoke declined by 54.2 mL/year. More importantly, all-cause mortality was significantly lower in the special intervention group than in the usual care group (8.83 per 1000 person-years vs. 10.38 per 1000 person-years; p=0.03).

It has been shown that repeated attempts to quit smoking, even with subsequent relapses, can prevent loss of lung function, especially in patients with mild COPD, and prolonged abstinence is also associated to a reduction in pulmonary symptoms. If a smoker with advanced COPD smoking, he/she will not recover lost lung function, but the subsequent rate of decline is likely to revert towards normal.

Smoking cessation at an early stage of the disease has shown to improve prognosis, and there is evidence that smoking cessation at an early stage of COPD is more effective than in the later stages. Smokers seem to be intrinsically more motivated to stop smoking if they realize that their respiratory complaints are caused by smoking and that they are at risk of developing COPD. In a recent study, smoking cessation rates were compared between smokers with COPD and smokers with normal lung function. During follow-up, the abstinence rates were significantly higher in smokers with COPD than in smokers with normal lung function.

Smoking Cessation Intervention Process.

Tobacco dependence is a chronic condition that often requires repeated intervention to succeed. Once users are dependent on tobacco, quitting is extremely difficult. Nicotine dependence resulting from tobacco use hinders efforts to sustain abstinence from tobacco for a prolonged period. Many users make multiple attempts to quit, often without the assistance that could significantly increase their chances of success. Studies have shown that a considerable number of smokers want to stop smoking, but a significant proportion of them have never tried. A large proportion of all smokers are in the stage of contemplation or the stage of preparation. Most smokers go through several stages before they finally take the decision to make a cessation attempt and at last succeed with their intentions and stop smoking. Smoking cessation advice or other interventions appear to have their effect by triggering a cessation attempt. Each year about 2% of smokers succeed in quitting on their own initiative.

Smoking cessation is challenging and behavioral interventions alone have had only modest success; as a result drug therapy has been increasingly relied upon to assist in smoking cessation. The most common of these pharmacologic interventions has been nicotine replacement therapy (NRT). More recently, attention has focused on the use of anti-depressant therapy. Pharmacologic smoking cessation aids are recommended for all smokers trying to quit, unless contraindicated;

Smokers should also be provided with counseling when attempting to quit. Family physicians can play an important role in the smoking cessation process, given that 70% of smokers consult family physicians annually.

As mentioned, most smokers who attempt to quit do not utilize cessation aids, and as a result, they are usually unsuccessful with two-thirds relapsing within 48 hours. For this reason, all smokers including those who may be at risk for COPD as well as those who already have the disease should be offered the most intensive smoking cessation intervention possible.

Genetic Considerations: Anti-trypsin Deficiency

Genetic factors can play an important role in the development of COPD. Of particular importance in this regard is A_1-antitrypsin (AAT), an enzyme that plays an important role in protecting against oxidative damage in the walls of the pulmonary alveoli and small bronchioles.

(AAT) deficiency was first described by Laurell and Eriksson in 1963. Laurell noted the absence of the band of alpha1- protein in 5 of 1500 serum protein electrophoreses (SPEP) submitted to his laboratory in Sweden. Laurell and Eriksson found that 3 out of the 5 patients had emphysema at young age, and that one had a family history of emphysema. Hence, the cardinal clinical features of AATD were established: absence of a protein in the alpha1 region of the SPEP, emphysema with early onset, and a genetic predisposition.

AAT is a protein normally found in the lungs and the bloodstream. It helps protect the lungs from the damage caused by inflammation that can lead to emphysema and chronic obstructive pulmonary disease (COPD). People whose bodies do not produce enough of this protein (AAT deficiency) are more likely to develop emphysema and to do so at a younger-than-normal age (30 to 40 years old). AAT deficiency is a rare disorder and is the only known genetic (inherited) factor that increases your risk of developing COPD.

Many genotypes expressing (AAT) exist and most individuals have high serum levels of (AAT). Consequently, genotypes expressing as (AAT) deficiencies can result in COPD in nonsmokers and can exacerbate the development of COPD in smokers. However, the role played by (AAT) deficiencies in COPD appears to be relatively minor given that severe (AAT) deficiencies occur in only 1-2% of COPD patients and COPD does not develop in all smokers with severe (AAT) deficiency.

The most common signs of lung disease in people with Alpha-1:
- Shortness of breath
- Wheezing
- Chronic cough and sputum (phlegm) production (chronic bronchitis)
- Recurring chest colds or pneumonia
- Low tolerance for exercise

- Non-responsive asthma or year-round allergies
- Bronchiectasis

Early diagnosis of Alpha-1 is very important because quitting smoking (if the Alpha smokes) and early treatment are both essential to help slow the progression of Alpha-1 lung disease. However, (AAT) deficiency can't be diagnosed by symptoms or by a medical examination alone; you need to get a blood test to know for sure. Alpha-1 is often first diagnosed as asthma or smoking-related Chronic Obstructive Pulmonary Disease (COPD). COPD includes emphysema and chronic bronchitis.

The Role of Air Pollution

Over the last 40 years, air pollution has increasingly been recognized as a significant causal factor in the development of some cases of COPD. An elevated prevalence of COPD has been noted in areas and cities where air pollution is high. Cigarette smoking is currently considered as the most important cause of COPD. However, cigarette smoking is not the sole cause for COPD. A recent study has shown that the population-attributable fraction for smoking as a cause of COPD ranged from 9.7% to 97.9%. The majority of population-attributable fraction estimates are less than 80%. In a Swedish cohort study with a 7-year follow-up (n = 963)7 involving subjects with objective lung function assessment for the diagnosis of COPD, a population-attributable fraction of 76.2% was found for smoking as a cause of COPD, whereas another cohort with 25-year follow-up in Denmark (n = 8045) reported a population attributable fraction of 74.6%. Like many other diseases, the development of COPD is multifactorial. Concerning the environmental factors, prolonged exposure to noxious particles and gases is related to the development of COPD. Traffic and other outdoor pollution, second-hand smoke and biomass smoke exposure are associated with COPD. However, there are currently insufficient criteria for a causation relationship.

Females regularly exposed to burning biomass commonly have obstructive airway disease and develop COPD with increased morbidity, with clinical characteristics and quality of life similar in degree to that of tobacco smokers. In addition, to playing an aetiological role in the genesis of COPD in some patients, there is now clear evidence that air pollution can induce exacerbations of airway obstruction COPD patients.

The APHEA study showed a relationship between emergency admissions for COPD and temporal trends in air pollution in European cities. Evidence from epidemiological studies have implicated air pollution, particularly black smoke, NO_2 and SO_2, in chronic respiratory symptoms and increased respiratory mortality in patients with COPD.

Reductions in respiratory mortality and morbidity were noted in COPD patients in Dublin following the introduction of legislation reducing the acceptable pollution levels from the burning bituminous coal.

The Role of Microbial Infections

COPD patients frequently demonstrate positive sputum culture to a variety of pathogenic bacteria, including *Streptococcus pneumonae, Haemophilus influenzae* and *Moraxella catarrhalis*. However, there is no clear evidence that respiratory infections are involved as aetiological or predisposing factors in the genesis of COPD. Nevertheless, there is abundant evidence that bacterial respiratory infections exacerbate airway obstruction and symptoms in COPD patients. The bacterial load in sputum is increased during exacerbations of COPD. In addition, *Streptococcus pneumonae, Haemophilus influenzae* and *Psuedomonas aeruginosa* have been shown to stimulate mucus hypersecretion *in vitro*. *Haemophilus influenzae* causes airway epithelial damage and *Haemophilus influenzae* endotoxin increases *in vitro* epithelial expression of the pro-inflammation cytokines TNF-a, IL-8, and IL-6.

Viral respiratory tract infections result in airway plasma exudation and the loss of ciliated airway epithelium and are a common precipitating factor in COPD exacerbations. Using cell and serology cultures, Gump *et al.*, (1976) proposed that 30% of COPD exacerbations are caused by viral infections. This compares with values of

40% - 50% of COPD exacerbations in studies that have utilized reverse transcriptase polymerase chain reactions.

The Natural History of COPD

Many smokers do not develop COPD, but a gradual progressive and irreversible decline in lung function occurs in susceptible persons while they continue to smoke. The FEV_1 will typically decline at a rate of 25-100 ml per year of smoking in susceptible people. In susceptible persons, COPD symptoms typically develop in the 5th decade of life as a result of many years of smoking, and disability from COPD typically commences in the 6th or 7th decade. The progression of COPD progressively affects quality of life as symptoms worsen and results in increased utilization of healthcare resources.

The development of COPD is variable between individuals, and not all patients follow the same clinical course. Some COPD patients have chronic phlegm and cough, whereas others primarily experience dyspnoea. In addition, some patients show an acute decline in lung function, whereas others experience a more chronic and slower reduction of function in lung function. After cessation of smoking, further progressive declines in FEV_1 return to the normal rate associated with ageing, but existing loss of FEV_1 is largely permanent. A small improvement in FEV_1 is sometimes observed within a year after cessation of smoking, compared with the accelerated rate of decline in those patients who continue to smoke.

Studies in the UK in the 1960s have shown that exacerbations of COPD were accompanied by a decline in respiratory function, but did not predict the rate of the progression of airflow obstruction. In addition, the progressive decline in FEV_1 did not respond to anticholinergic drugs therapy or by the use of inhaled steroids. Sputum production, symptoms of cough, dyspnoea and history of exposure to risk factors are important considerations in the diagnosis of COPD. Most COPD patients who develop breathlessness will visit their family doctor. Consequently, it is not surprising the dyspnoea and cough are described as initial symptoms by the majority of COPD patients with moderate airflow obstruction in both North America and. A United Kingdom study has reported chronic bronchitis, sputum production and symptoms of cough in 7% of women and 17% of men with chronic bronchitis who smoked aged 40 years old or older. In a more recent and extensive study from the USA, 12.5% of current smokers had airflow obstruction and 25% of male smoker suffered from chronic cough.

Pathophysiology of COPD

Chronic inflammatory processes result in small airways disease in COPD patients. These inflammatory processes are not fully understood and respond poorly to current pharmacological treatment. During exacerbations of COPD airway inflammation worsens with resultant pathophysiological deterioration and accompanying symptoms. These events result in increased airway secretions and airway narrowing, with excess sputum, increased dyspnoea and cough. Airway inflammatory markers such as neutrophils and interleukin (IL-6 and IL-8) are elevated in sputum from COPD patients. In addition, elevated numbers of inflammatory cells such as eosinophils and neutrophils have been reported in airway biopsies, bronchoalveolar lavage and induced sputum in patients during exacerbations of COPD.

The National Institute of Health Intermittent Positive Pressure Breathing trial carried out extensive post mortem studies into COPD and showed that most patients dying of COPD had both extensive airway inflammation and emphysema. Severe COPD exacerbations also result in hypoxemia with or without hypercapnia. The pathophysiologic events which connect the symptoms of COPD exacerbations to respiratory failure to airway inflammation are outlined in Figure (18).

Understanding the natural history of COPD is dependent on assessing whether lung function deteriorates over time in different individuals such as non-susceptible smokers, susceptible smokers, and nonsmokers. However, measurements of lung function are variable even when repeated daily or during the same test session and measured changes depend on the reproducibility of pre- and post-bronchodilator results.

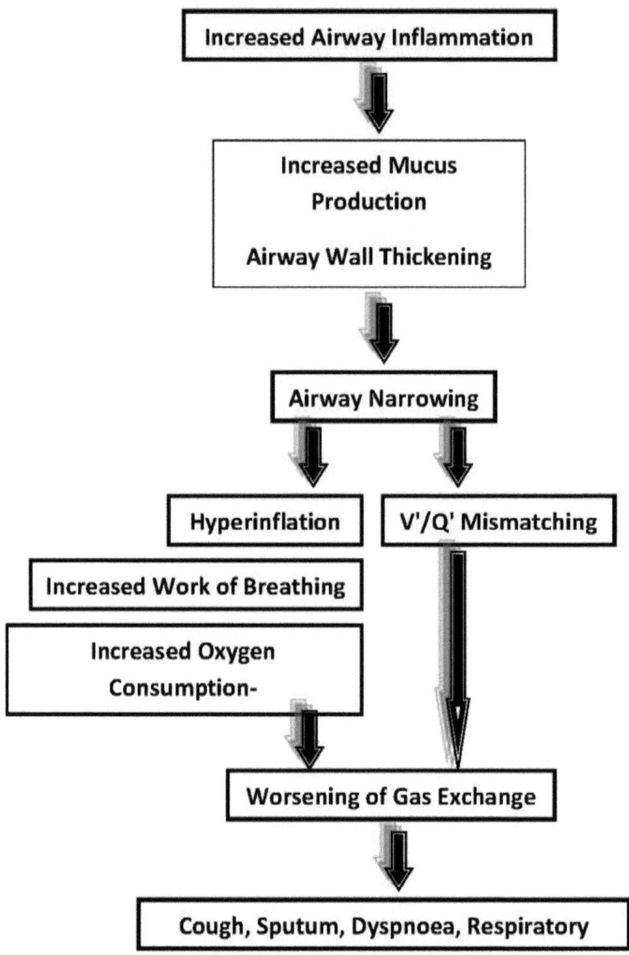

Fig 18. Schematic presentation of the main pathophysiologic events of COPD exacerbations, starting from increased airway inflammation.

The FEV1 is considered an important repeatable lung function parameter with short term changes of > 0.2 L and 12% often being clinically significant. Spirometric measurement of maximum expiratory airflows such as the FEV1 is useful when assessing the respiratory pathophysiological status of COPD patients and is routinely used for this purpose. A FEV1 to forced vital capacity ratio of <70% is used in the present ATS/ERS and GOLD definition for airflow limitation.

The value of forced expiratory tests such as the FEV1 is based on the following considerations. Airway obstruction in COPD manifests itself predominantly during the expiratory phase of breathing when the pressure surrounding the intrapulmonary airways exceeds the intraluminal airway pressure and causes these airways to become dynamically compressed in a manner akin to a Starling resistor. Under such conditions, a state of effort independent expiratory airflow limitation is said to exist because increases in expiratory effort act to further the degree of dynamic airway compression and hence further impede expiratory airflow. In mild cases of COPD, expiratory airflow limitation is only evident during high expiratory airflows which require high levels of expiratory effort. However, expiratory airflow limitation occurs at progressively lower levels of expiratory airflow as COPD becomes more severe. Eventually, a stage is reached in severe COPD cases where expiratory airflow limitation occurs during quiet tidal
Breathing and causing the patient to irreversibly gasp for every breath even under resting conditions.

The lungs are typically hyperinflated in COPD patients and this is evident on physical examination an on chest radiographs. Several factors contribute to pulmonary hyperinflation in COPD. First, increased airflow obstruction during the expiratory phase of breathing ensures that lung volume fails to fall to its normal relaxation volume at end expiration resulting in what is termed dynamic pulmonary hyperinflation. The degree of dynamic pulmonary hyperinflation increases as airflow obstruction worsens or when minute ventilation (VE) increases so that there is insufficient time for the lungs to deflate to their end-expiratory relaxation volume. In addition, significant closure of small airways occurs in COPD and the resultant air trapping behind such closed airways contributes to pulmonary hyperinflation in these patients. The volume of air trapping and the resultant pulmonary hyperinflation increases as COPD worsens.

Lung Pathology in COPD

A variety of pathological changes occur in the airway and alveolar walls as a result of the ongoing inflammatory processes within the lungs of COPD patients. Histological changes resulting from chronic airway inflammation that contribute to airway narrowing in COPD include: hypertrophy of airway smooth muscle, fibrosis in the bronchiolar wall, metaplasia of mucous secreting goblet cells, enlargement of mucous glands and squamous metaplasia of the airway mucosa which impairs mucociliary clearance. The pulmonary alveoli also frequently undergo pathological changes in COPD with destruction of the alveolar walls and enlargement of the alveoli. Emphysematous changes can also result in macroscopic collections of air in the lungs called bullae and intrapulmonary bronchogenic cysts, and in the intrapleural space (blebs).

Epidemiology of COPD

Most epidemiological data on COPD comes from industrialised countries that have extensive and well-resourced health systems and regularly carry out extensive health surveys. It is also important to note that substantial international differences in COPD epidemiology exist, and that revisions and international differences in the definition of COPD can impede analysis of epidemiological data.

Prevalence

There is unanimous agreement within the medical community that increases in cigarette smoking have led to increases in COPD prevalence globally. Data from unpublished and published sources analyzed by the Global Burden of Disease study which have been undertaken with the full collaboration and participation of the World

Health Organization and the World Bank, concluded that there was a global increase in the prevalence of COPD at a rate just under 1% over 4.5 years. However, large differences in COPD prevalence exist in different countries. Using symptoms of airflow limitation, the Nutrition Examination Survey and The National Health Service in the USA estimated that COPD prevalence was around 14% for current smokers in the USA between 1988 and 1994.

Another study conducted by the UK General Practice Research Database used physician-based diagnosis in 50714 patients, and reported a prevalence rate increased from 0.80% in 1990 to 1.36% in 1997 in females for all ages and 1.35% to 1.65% for males.

Hospitalization Admission Rates

Hospital admission records provide an additional useful source of epidemiological data. In a longitudinal study in Cleveland USA, Rita *et al.* (1997) reported an increase in patients hospitalized for COPD from 162,899 in 1984 to 131,974 in 1991. In addition, since the early 1990s, the number of admissions to hospital for COPD has steadily increased in England. Between 1998 and 2003, the English Department of Health reported that the number of hospital admissions for COPD had increased by 13.1%. During 2003 to 2004, COPD was responsible for more than 2.4% of the 4.2 million acute medical admissions and 0.9% of all 11.7 million hospital admission in England.

A Danish study using 876 randomly selected males from the national Hospital Discharge Register reported that respiratory symptoms and FEV_1 were both powerful predictors of hospitalization for COPD. It is not clear whether these male findings also apply to female COPD patients. However, Prescott *et al.* (1997) have argued that there is no reason to assume that females COPD patients are admitted to hospital more readily than males COPD patients.

Severity

Substantial differences in COPD severity have been reported in different countries. Zielinski *et al*. (2006) conducted an epidemiological study on COPD severity in Italy using GOLD criteria, and chronic respiratory failure requiring long-term oxygen therapy and the presence of moderate to severe airway obstruction, as criteria of severe COPD. There workers reported that severe to very severe, moderate and mild COPD was present in 0.3%, 2.2% and 7.3% of adult females respectively, and in 0.4, 4.5% and 12.3% of adult males, respectively. In another European study (Italy), 3% of COPD patients were severely affected and 26% were moderately affected.

The epidemiological survey reported similar findings in Northern Sweden. In contrast, the rate of severe COPD in both Norway and Sweden was found to be <1% in the 1970s and 1990s, while in the USA severe COPD occurred in 1.7% of the general population during this period. In addition, a Copenhagen survey, reported that 0.2% of adults had severe COPD and 5.2% had moderate COPD.

Morbidity

The USA National Health Interview study and National Center Health Statistics of 1971-2000 estimated that around 10 million men and women had COPD. This compares with an earlier USA study carried out by Tecumseh and Michigan Community Health which surveyed over 4,499 women and men in 1973 and reported that around 8% of adult women and 14% of adult men have obstructive airway disease, chronic bronchitis, or both. Survey assessment of physician diagnosis rates in 1,003 patients with COPD in the United States in 2006 indicated that 61% of patients reported moderate or severe dyspnoea and that 41% reported prior hospitalization for COPD.

The most prevalent comorbid diagnoses were hypertension (55%), hypercholesterolemia (52%), depression (37%), cataracts (31%) and osteoporosis (28%). In the USA, both mortality and frequency of hospitalizations of COPD patients were accompanied by several comorbidities such as diabetes, ischemic heart disease, hypertension, chronic heart failure, pneumonia, respiratory failure, thoracic malignancy, and pulmonary vascular disease.

Mortality

Mortality rates for COPD vary substantially in different countries. In addition, mortality from COPD is frequently associated with other comorbidities, and many patients with COPD die after suffering from other disabilities and dyspnoea. This can complicate estimates of mortality directly attributable to COPD. Nevertheless, COPD is regarded as the fourth leading cause of death in the world, responsible for about 4.8% of deaths annually, which translates to some 2.75 million deaths annually worldwide. In another study, it was estimated that 600 million people suffer from COPD which accounted for 2.5 million deaths in 2000.

In Romania and the Ukraine, COPD accounts for up to 80 deaths per 100,000 population, whereas in Iceland, Greece, Norway, and Sweden COPD deaths results in approximately <20 deaths per 100,000 population. High mortality rates from COPD have also been reported in Wales and England, as shown below in **Figure 19**. In France, COPD was the main cause of death which was analyzed with the underlying causes (Fuhrman *et al.*, 2006), with mortality rate from COPD of 40 deaths per 100,000 populations.

Mortality rates from COPD have been shown to increase in conjunction with increased cigarette consumption in developing countries such as in China where cigarette smoking causes approximately 12% of all deaths. By 2020, it is has been predicted that COPD will be the third main cause of death worldwide. However, it is significant to note that many of these deaths are potentially preventable because mortality from COPD decreases following cessation of smoking. Mortality from COPD correlates with the severity of the disease and with age in people over 45 years old, and this applies especially in males.

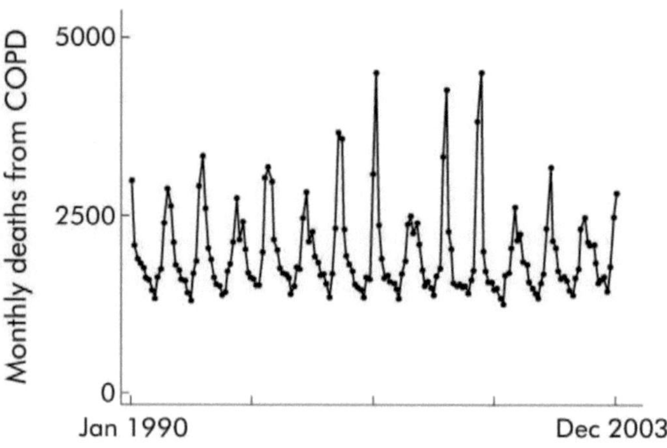

Fig 19. Monthly deaths from COPD (ICD9 490–492 and 496 for years before 2001 and ICD10 J40–J44 thereafter) at any age for men and women living in England and Wales. To be compatible with deaths in 1990–1992, data for the years from 1993 were divided by 0.920 to adjust for differences in coding instructions; deaths for 2001–2003 were then divided by 0.966 to allow for differences between ICD9 and ICD10. Data from the UK Office of National Statistics.

A number of studies have examined pre-bronchodilator FEV_1 and bronchodilator response as potential predictors of mortality in COPD, but have reported conflicting results. In other studies, spirometric assessment including the FEV_1, the body mass index (BMI) and dyspnoea are regarded as important predictors of mortality and health status in COPD. In addition, indices incorporating the 6-min walk test, nutritional status (body mass index), severity of obstructive airflow, and the severity of dyspnoea appear to predict COPD mortality better than FEV_1 alone.

Effects of Burden and Costs of COPD on the Health System

COPD imposes an enormous burden on healthcare systems and society. The cost per patient increases with COPD severity, as was demonstrated in Spain where the cost per patient with moderate to mild COPD was three to seven times less than that for patients with severe COPD. In Sweden, the costs of hospitalization for COPD patients in 1999 were evaluated of USD 871 million, patients with moderate disease (13%) accounted for 41%, whereas patients with mild disease (83%) accounted for 29% of the total costs. The patients with severe disease (4%) accounted for the remainder (30%).

In Italy, the cost per patient with severe COPD was estimated to cost € 6366 and € 1861 respectively in year, whereas in Denmark for 1998-2002, the costs related to hospitalization of COPD patients was estimated to be € 256 million. The French SCOPE study estimated the total medical resource consumption costs of a COPD patient per year to be about € 4,366. One quarter of the French costs was due to complications related to COPD (mainly exacerbations) and one-third of the costs was related to hospitalizations. In the Netherlands, the yearly costs of COPD were estimated to be € 813 per patient in year.

The costs related to COPD are likely to increase markedly in the future. **Figure 20** shows the total predicted costs of COPD by 2015 compared with 1994. Two estimates of future costs are given for the total population and for women and men separately. Both estimates assume stable costs per patient; the first includes changes in smoking behavior, and the second assumes constant incidence rates. It is estimated that from 1994 to 2015 that total costs will increase over 90%, and that the cost increase is expected to be less for men than women because of normal baseline mortality rates.

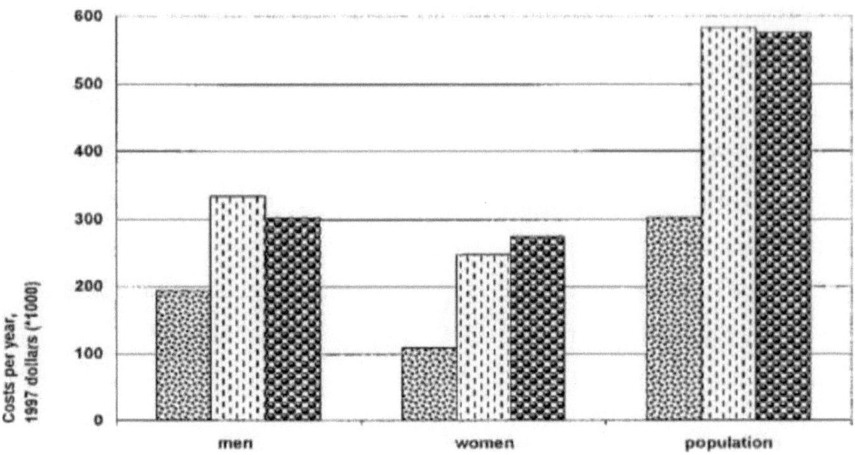

Fig 20. COPD costs of care at constant treatment patterns in 1994 and projections for 2015 for male, female and total population. *First bar* from left in each group of three _ 1994 level, *middle bar* in each group of three _ 2015, projection at constant incidence rates; *third bar* from left in each group of three _ 2015, projection including changes in smoking behavior.

Dyspnoea in COPD

Dyspnoea is an unpleasant sensation of breathlessness (Mahler *et al.*, 1992) and is a consequence of varied and complex interactions. Dyspnoea has been defined as *"a subjective experience of breathing discomfort that consists of qualitatively distinct sensations that vary in intensity. The experience derives from interactions among multiple physiological, psychological, social, and environmental factors, and may induce secondary physiological and behavioural responses"*.

Dyspnoea or breathlessness is a hallmark symptom in COPD. It occurs early in COPD and progressively worsens as the severity of COPD advances so that patients are normally breathless on minimal exertion by the time that the FEV_1 has fallen to below 30% of the predicted levels. The worsening dyspnoea and ongoing loss of exercise tolerance progressively impairs the COPD patient's quality of life.

Dyspnea is the term generally applied to sensations experienced by individuals who complain of unpleasant or uncomfortable respiratory sensations. Many definitions of dyspnea have been offered, including: "difficult, labored, uncomfortable breathing", an "awareness of respiratory distress", "the sensation of feeling breathless or experiencing air hunger", and "an uncomfortable sensation of breathing". These definitions have sometimes mixed the true symptom (what patients say they are feeling) with physical signs (what the physician observes about the patient, e.g., "exhibits labored breathing"). In the final analysis, a symptom can only be described by the person who experiences it. In this context, recent investigations of the perception of breathlessness suggest that there are multiple types of dyspnea. Given our greater understanding of the interplay between physiological and behavioral factors in producing respiratory discomfort as well as the spectrum of phrases used by patients to describe their sensations, we propose a broader definition of dyspnea. Specifically, we suggest that dyspnea is a term used to characterize a subjective experience of breathing discomfort that consists of qualitatively distinct sensations that vary in intensity. The experience derives from interactions among multiple physiological, psychological, social, and environmental factors, and may induce secondary physiological and behavioral responses. This broad definition of dyspnea will guide our discussion.

Mechanisms of Dyspnoea

A variety of mechanisms are believed to be involved in the generation of dyspnoea. A wide range of sensory inputs are believed to contribute to dyspnoea in various disease states. Such sensory inputs can arise from stimulation of afferents in the airway wall, lung parenchyma, and around pulmonary capillaries (i.e. airway irritant receptors, Paintball's juxtapulmonary J receptors), chemoreceptors, tendon organs, muscle spindles, joint and skin receptors.

It has been known since the classic study by Marshall *et al.* (1954) that increased respiratory effort and mechanical power can result in dyspnoea. Increased respiratory effort can result from a variety of reasons, including increased minute ventilation, increased respiratory resistive load and increased elastic respiratory loads. Increased respiratory drive can result in dyspnoea, in part because the work and effort of breathing are increased.

Hypoxemia, hypercapnia, and acidosis can lead to air hunger and thereby play important roles in the generation of dyspnoea. Impaired inspiratory muscle function can also contribute to the genesis of dyspnoea, and such impaired muscle function may be due to muscle atrophy and sub-optimal inspiratory muscle length during lung hyperinflation. In addition, anxiety and depression result in increased severity of dyspnoea and adversely affect quality of life in patients with COPD. Thus, the patient's emotional state can exert important influences on the expression of respiratory sensations and thereby alter the quality and severity of dyspnoea.

Campbell and his friends coined the term "length-tension inappropriateness" to describe an abnormal relationship between the respiratory muscle motor command and the resulting mechanical response of the respiratory system, which is then sensed as respiratory discomfort. More recently, a "neuro-mechanical" model of dyspnoea has emerged which includes not only information arising from the ventilatory muscles, but also information arising from receptors throughout the respiratory system.

The sensation of dyspnea seems to originate with the activation of sensory systems involved with respiration. Sensory information is, in turn, relayed to higher brain centers where central processing of respiratory-related signals and contextual, cognitive, and behavioral influences shape the ultimate expression of the evoked sensation. The homeostatic systems involved in the regulation of respiration provide a framework for understanding the mechanisms of dyspnea.

Physiological Mechanisms

Our understanding of the physiologic mechanisms underlying the sensations of dyspnea is derived from studies employing a range of experimental conditions in animals, normal subjects, anesthetized subjects, and patients with cardiopulmonary and neurologic diseases. Conclusions from these findings, and apparent contradictions among studies, must be viewed with an appreciation for the fact that those species differences and, in man, state differences, may have powerful effects on respiratory phenomena.

Respiratory motor command corollary discharge

There is a conscious awareness of the outgoing respiratory motor command to the ventilatory muscles. This sense of respiratory motor output is distinct from sensations directly related to changes in muscle length or tension and is attributed to a corollary discharge from brainstem respiratory neurons to the sensory cortex during automatic reflex breathing or from cortical motor centers to the sensory cortex during voluntary respiratory efforts. Evidence for corollary discharges is functional rather than structural; specific receptors and pathways have not been identified. However, rostral projections from brainstem respiratory motor neurons to the midbrain and thalamus have recently been described in the cat, and these could represent the pathway of corollary discharges. These corollary discharges are thought to be important in shaping the sense of respiratory effort. It is well established
that factors that necessitate a greater motor command to achieve a given tension in the muscle, such as decreasing muscle length, muscle fatigue, or respiratory muscle weakness, cause a heightened sense of respiratory effort. The sense of respiratory effort intensifies with increases in central respiratory motor command and is proportional to the ratio of the pressures generated by the respiratory muscles to the maximum pressure–generating capacity of those muscles.

Chest wall receptors

Projections to the brain of afferent signals from mechanoreceptors in the joints, tendons, and muscles of the chest all appear to play a role in shaping respiratory sensations. Specifically, afferents from intercostal muscles have been shown to project to the cerebral cortex and contribute to proprioception and kinesthesia. Studies of the detection of just noticeable differences in added external ventilatory loads have suggested a primary role for muscle spindles in mediating the sensation of dyspnea. The sentience of chest wall muscles is further supported by the observations that vibration of the chest wall to activate muscle spindles produces an illusion of chest movement.

Vibration of inspiratory muscles located in the upper rib cage in phase with inspiration produces a sensation of chest expansion and reduces the intensity of dyspnea in patients with chronic lung disease, both at rest and during exercise. Voluntarily constraining ventilation (E) below the spontaneously adopted breathing level produces an intense sensation of air hunger, even when blood gases and the chemical drive to breathe are not allowed to change. The increase in the intensity of dyspnea associated with reduced ventilation at a constant PCO2 correlates closely with the degree to which tidal volume is reduced. This effect of constrained thoracic expansion on respiratory sensation is modified by chest wall vibration; with vibration of the upper rib cage during inspiration, the intensity of dyspnea associated with constrained
breathing is reduced, suggesting a preeminent role for chest wall receptors.

Pulmonary vagal receptors

Afferent information from pulmonary vagal receptors project to the brain, and vagal inputs are important in shaping the pattern of breathing. There is some evidence that vagal influences, independent of any effect on the level and pattern of breathing, may also contribute to the sensation of dyspnea. Patients with high cervical spinal cord transection, in whom feedback from chest wall receptors is blocked, are able to detect changes in tidal volume delivered by a mechanical ventilator, and experience a sensation of air hunger when their in-V spired volume is reduced. This suggests that vagal receptors may contribute to the unpleasant sensations that result when thoracic expansion is limited and to the dyspnea that accompanies breath holding. Additionally, it has been shown that vagal blockade ameliorates dyspnea during exercise and alleviates the unpleasant sensations during breath holding. Dyspnea associated with bronchoconstriction is at least in part mediated by vagal afferents. This is suggested by the observation that the heightened sensation of difficulty in breathing resulting from airway obstruction induced by histamine inhalation is lessened following the inhalation of lidocaine to block airway receptors. Other studies have shown the intravenous injections of lobe line to stimulate pulmonary C fibers produces a sensation of choking and pressure in the chest.

Chemoreceptors

The dyspnea associated with hypercapnia and hypoxia is largely the result of the chemically induced increases in respiratory motor activity. There is some evidence that the sensation of dyspnea may also be directly affected by inputs from chemoreceptors. Both ventilator-dependent quadriplegics with high cervical spinal cord transection and normal subjects paralyzed with neuromuscular blocking agents experience sensations of air hunger when PCO_2 is increased. Also, the sensation of dyspnea is more intense at given levels of ventilation produced by hypercapnia compared to the same level of ventilation achieved by exercise or by voluntary hyperventilation. It has also been shown that the relief of exercise-induced hypoxemia by the administration of oxygen results in a reduction of dyspnea out of proportion to the reduction in ventilation.

Pathophysiology of Dyspnea

An attractive unifying theory is that dyspnea results from a disassociation or a mismatch between central respiratory motor activity and incoming afferent information from receptors in the airways, lungs, and chest wall structures. The afferent feedback from peripheral sensory receptors may allow the brain to assess the effectiveness of the motor commands issued to the ventilatory muscles, i.e., the appropriateness of the response in terms of flow and volume for the command. When changes in respiratory pressure, airflow, or movement

of the lung and chest wall are not appropriate for the outgoing motor command, the intensity of dyspnea is heightened. In other words, a dissociation between the motor command and the mechanical response of the respiratory system may produce a sensation of respiratory discomfort. This mechanism was first introduced by Campbell and Howell in the 1960s with the theory of "length-tension inappropriateness." The theory has been generalized to include not only information arising in the ventilatory muscles, but information emanating from receptors throughout the respiratory system and has been termed "neuro-mechanical", or "efferent–reafferent dissociation". Patients with a mechanical load on the respiratory system, either resistive or elastic, or respiratory muscle abnormalities will have a dissociation between the efferent and afferent information during breathing. The mismatch of neural activity and consequent mechanical or ventilator outputs may contribute to the intensity of dyspnea under these conditions. This theory explains dyspnea associated with breath holding, the unpleasant sensation of air hunger experienced by patients receiving mechanical ventilation with small tidal volumes and low inspiratory flow rates, and the discomfort of subjects who voluntarily constrain the rate and depth of their breathing. Heightened ventilatory demand. It is regularly observed, both in normal individuals and in patients with lung disease, that the intensity of the dyspnea increases progressively with the level of ventilation during exercise. This is attributable to the increase in respiratory motor output and a corresponding increase in the sense of effort. There are, however, important contextual influences on the interpretation of respiratory- related sensations. Thus, symptoms of shortness of breath are more likely to be reported when hyperpnea occurs at rest and cannot be accounted for by an increase in exertion or physical activity. Many conditions give rise to ventilation that is excessive for the level of physical activity, and consequently cause symptoms of dyspnea. Increases in ventilation are required to compensate for the enlarged dead space that results from lung parenchymal and pulmonary vascular disease. Hypoxemia at altitude and in patients with respiratory disease stimulates arterial chemoreceptors and increases respiratory motor activity.

This heightened motor command contributes to dyspnea. Patients with cardiorespiratory disease are often deconditioned because of prolonged inactivity. The state of physical conditioning is an important determinant of exercise capacity. Deconditioning is associated with an early and accelerated rise in blood lactate levels. Early lactic acid production by skeletal muscles during exercise imposes an additional respiratory stimulus, increases the ventilation at a given level of exercise, and heightens dyspnea. This and the additional burdens of advanced age, malnutrition, and hypoxemia impair respiratory and peripheral muscle function and lead to limitations in exercise capacity secondary to leg discomfort and dyspnea. The cycle of dyspnea, reduced activity, deconditioning, and more dyspnea is well recognized as a key contributor to the functional decline associated with both normal aging and cardiorespiratory illness.

While the level of ventilation often correlates well with the intensity of dyspnea, increases in central inspiratory activity alone are unlikely to explain respiratory discomfort in all settings. As noted previously, for a given level of ventilation, different stimuli produce dyspnea of varying intensity, and supplemental oxygen reduces dyspnea associated with exercise in hypoxic subjects out of proportion to the reduction in ventilation. In addition, if all dyspnea were the consequence of heightened ventilatory demand, one might expect the quality of respiratory discomfort to be similar in all situations, a hypothesis that is unable to account for the findings of recent studies on the language of dyspnea, in which patients with different pathophysiologic conditions characterize their discomfort utilizing qualitatively distinct phrases.

Respiratory muscle abnormalities

Weakness or mechanical inefficiency of the respiratory muscles results in a mismatch between central respiratory motor output and achieved ventilation. This mismatch may explain the dyspnea experienced by patients with neuromuscular diseases affecting the respiratory musculature and patients with respiratory muscle fatigue. As the pressure-generating capacity of the respiratory muscles fall and as the ratio of the pressures produced by the respiratory muscles to the maximum pressure that can be achieved increases, dyspnea progressively worsens.

Chronic obstructive pulmonary disease (COPD) is often characterized by overinflation of the lung and overexpansion of the thorax. This results in an enlarged FRC and foreshortening of the muscles of inspiration. Based on the length–tension properties of muscle, foreshortening of the inspiratory muscles in COPD may substantially reduce their force-generating capacity. This impairment in the mechanical advantage of the inspiratory muscles contributes importantly to symptoms of dyspnea. The relief of dyspnea following lung volume reduction surgery may be explained, at least in part, by the resulting changes in thoracic size and shape with increases in the resting length of the muscles of inspiration. Airflow limitation in patients with COPD leads to dynamic hyperinflation, particularly during exercise. Several important consequences of dynamic hyperinflation serve to worsen dyspnea. The increase in lung volume causes breathing to take

place on a stiffer portion of the pressure–volume curve, producing an added elastic load. The inward elastic recoil of the respiratory system at end-expiration imposes an added inspiratory threshold load. Finally, inspiratory muscle shortening with hyperinflation reduces muscle mechanical efficiency. The relief of dyspnea with inhaled bronchodilators has been attributed to reductions in exercise dynamic hyperinflation.

Abnormal ventilatory impedance

Respiratory diseases such as asthma and COPD which narrow airways and increase airway resistance, and diseases of the lung parenchyma, including interstitial pneumonitis and pulmonary fibrosis, which increase lung elastance, commonly cause dyspnea. When ventilator impedance increases, the level of central respiratory motor output required to achieve a given ventilation rises. When the respiratory effort expended in breathing is out of proportion to the resulting level of ventilation, dyspnea results.

Changes in ventilatory impedance produced by diseases of the lungs can be simulated in normal subjects by the imposition of external ventilatory resistive and elastic loads. As the magnitude of the applied external ventilatory load is increased, there is a progressive rise in the intensity of dyspnea. Dyspnea intensity during external ventilatory loading corresponds primarily to the peak airway pressures developed by the contracting respiratory muscles, the duration of inspiration, and the breathing frequency.

Abnormal breathing patterns

Dyspnea is common in diseases involving the lung parenchyma. It is possible that the rapid shallow breathing often noted in diseases of the lung parenchyma is a reflex response to the stimulation of pulmonary vagal receptors, but there is little direct evidence that pulmonary vagal receptors contribute directly to dyspnea. Pulmonary vagal receptors have been posited to play a role in the dyspnea of severe exercise, pulmonary congestion and pulmonary edema, and recurrent pulmonary embolism. Pursed lip breathing has been associated with reduced dyspnea intensity in patients with obstructive lung disease, an effect that may be due to a diminished respiratory frequency, changes in the pattern of ventilatory muscle recruitment, longer expiratory time, and larger tidal volumes.

Blood-gas abnormalities

Blood-gas abnormalities, while among the most serious consequences of cardiorespiratory disease, poorly correlate with dyspnea in individual patients. Hypoxemia causes respiratory motor activity to increase through chemoreceptor stimulation. Hypoxia may also have a direct dyspnogenic effect. This is suggested by the observation that supplemental oxygen administration relieves dyspnea in some patients with lung disease, even in the absence of any changes in ventilation. Similarly, the dyspnea produced by hypercapnia is largely the consequence of increases in respiratory motor output, but there also appears to be a direct effect of PCO2 on the intensity of dyspnea. The effect of PCO2 on ventilation depends primarily on changes in hydrogen ion concentration at the medullary chemoreceptors. In patients with chronic hypercapnia, metabolic compensation minimizes any changes in hydrogen ion concentration and consequently limits ventilatory responses and changes in respiratory sensation. On the other hand, the responses to changes in hydrogen ion concentration may explain the dyspnea of diabetic ketoacidosis and renal insufficiency.

Qualities of Dyspnea and Physiologic Mechanisms

Utilizing dyspnea questionnaires in three studies involving more than 300 patients with a variety of cardiopulmonary disorders, both in the United States and the United Kingdom, investigators have demonstrated that individuals with presumed different physiologic causes for their breathing discomfort, as well as normal subjects made breathless by performing a variety of respiratory tasks, employ qualitatively distinct sensations to describe that discomfort. While the sense of increased effort or work of breathing is a common feature for conditions characterized by abnormal mechanical loads (e.g., COPD, interstitial lung disease) and neuromuscular weakness, patients with congestive heart failure described a sensation of air hunger or suffocating, and the dyspnea of asthma is notable for a sensation of chest tightness. The consistency of these findings across a large number of patients in two different cultures suggests that

these qualities of dyspnea reflect not merely variations in individual expectations or experiences,
but inherent differences in the physiologic mechanisms underlying the sensations themselves.

Several studies have begun to provide additional direct information on the relationship between quality of dyspnea and the underlying mechanism producing discomfort. The sensation of air hunger has been shown to be associated with increases in respiratory drive, particularly in the presence of hypoxia or hypercapnia. While the intensity of this sensation may be modified by changes in tidal volume, changes that are likely to be sensed in part by transmission of afferent information from pulmonary stretch receptors to the central nervous system, the basic quality of the sensation persists. Furthermore, in an experimental model in which normal subjects were asked to breathe at a targeted level of hyperpnoea while $PaCO_2$ was modified by varying the concentration of inspired carbon dioxide, subjects were able to independently rate their sense of effort to breathe and sense of air hunger or unpleasant urge to breathe (80). As $PaCO_2$ was raised, air hunger increased while the effort of breathing decreased.

These data are consistent with the notion that the sensation of air hunger is associated with stimulation of chemoreceptors while the sense of effort to breathe may reflect central respiratory motor command (37). In studies of methacholine-induced bronchoconstriction in subjects with mild asthma, several sensations of breathing discomfort appear in a sequential fashion. At very mild degrees of airway obstruction, the sensation of chest tightness predominates. As FEV1 falls and the mechanical load on the system increases, the sensation of effort emerges while further declines in lung function are associated with a sensation of air hunger. These findings suggest that chest tightness may arise from bronchoconstriction-induced stimulation of pulmonary receptors, while the sensation of effort reflects the increased central motor command associated with the worsening mechanical load on the system. Air hunger may emerge in concert with even greater central motor activity. In patients with asthma presenting to an emergency department with acute flares of their disease, inhaled b-agonists reduce the sensation of chest tightness, while the effort and work of breathing, along with airways obstruction, persist. Thus, induction of bronchoconstriction produces chest tightness; alleviation of bronchoconstriction eliminates it. To the extent that airway inflammation, airways obstruction, and mechanical load persist, the sense of effort remains.

Measuring Dyspnoea

Dyspnoea severity is routinely carried out to diagnose COPD and to assess the severity of impairment. A variety of techniques are used to evaluate the severity of dyspnoea. Instruments such as the Visual Analogue Scale (VAS) and Borg Category Scale are used to measure current perceived dyspnoea by asking the subject to mentally quantify and communicate the intensity of the dyspnoea.

A variety of questionnaire based approaches are used to evaluate dyspnoea, over relatively prolonged recent periods (e.g. several weeks) and assess the contribution that dyspnoea makes to the patient's sense of wellbeing during activities of daily living (ADL). Such questionnaire based instruments explore a range of aspects relating to dyspnoea, and include the modified the Health Related Quality of Life (HRQoL) questionnaire, modified Medical Research Council (MRC) Dyspnoea Scale, the Baseline Dyspnoea Index (BDI), the Chronic Respiratory Disease Questionnaire (CRQ) and the St. George's Respiratory Questionnaire (SGRQ).

The MRC consists of a brief questionnaire that assesses the workload required to precipitate dyspnoea during walking. The BDI is a more complex instrument that grades impairment arising from dyspnoea in each of five separate categories: functional impairment, magnitude of task, and magnitude of effort grades of impairment relating to each of the following categories. The CRQ grades impairment arising from dyspnoea in each of three separate components. Similarly, the SGRQ grades impairment arising from dyspnoea in each of three separate categories: those concerned with respiratory symptoms, activities that are limited by dyspnoea, and the overall disturbance to the patient (Jones et al., 1992). In addition, questionnaire based instruments such as the HRQoL are also available that assess the impact of dyspnoea on various domains of the patient's quality of life.

Hajiro and colleagues (1998) investigated the relationships between different measures of dyspnoea in COPD patients. These workers examined clinical dyspnoea ratings (e.g. MRC, BDI), the influence of dyspnoea on HRQoL using a disease-specific questionnaire such as the St. George's Respiratory Questionnaire (SGRQ) and the Chronic Respiratory Disease Questionnaire (CRQ), and dyspnoea during maximal exercise using the Borg Scale. Clinical dyspnoea ratings and dimensions of the disease-specific HRQoL questionnaires gave similar dyspnoea ratings. In contrast, the Borg scale dyspnoea ratings did not correlate closely with the clinical dyspnoea ratings or the HRQoL, possibly because the Borg scale evaluated a different aspect of dysponea under the exercise conditions of the study.

The MRC Dyspnoea Scale has also been used to explore the relationships between dyspnoea severity, exercise tolerance, health status, activities of daily living, and lung function in COPD patients.

Chapter Four

Function and Training of the Respiratory Muscles in COPD

The respiratory muscles are skeletal muscles that power the vital function of pulmonary ventilation. Many COPD patients have impaired respiratory muscle function which has a significant adverse effect on their lives. Impairment of inspiratory muscle function is of particular importance in COPD patients. Skeletal muscle function is frequently impaired in patients with COPD, even in those persons affected by mild disease. Whether the abnormalities are mainly due to deconditioning are more related to a systemic effect of the disease, or, indeed, result from its treatment with corticosteroids is still a matter for discussion. The main abnormalities that are described are skeletal muscle weakness, atrophy, muscle damage, excessive cell death by apoptosis, and myopathy. Muscle weakness is associated with significant disability and can affect the overall prognosis. First, muscle weakness contributes to exercise intolerance in COPD. Second, patients with frequent hospital admissions show a greater degree of impairment of muscle strength than do patients who make less use of health care resources. Finally, patients with steroid-induced myopathy have a reduced survival rate. Recently, is shown that reduced muscle bulk, as measured by mid-thigh cross sectional area, is an important contributor to survival, even in patients with moderate COPD. These observations suggest that reversing skeletal muscle weakness should be a target of therapy for COPD. However, two treatment types are currently available for impaired inspiratory muscle function in COPD patients: inspiratory muscle training and surgery (lung transplantation and lung volume reduction surgery).

Pulmonary rehabilitation utilizes inspiratory muscle training. Meta-analysis of training regimes for patients with COPD shows the benefits of inspiratory muscle training. A controlled randomized study of 30 patients with COPD supported the use of inspiratory muscle training and participants showed an increase in maximal inspiratory pressure. Whereas, the palliation of dyspnoea in advanced COPD patients is treated by transplantation and lung volume reduction surgery.

The inspiratory muscle strength and endurance are significantly increased after inspiratory muscle training. In addition, inspiratory muscle training induced structural changes within the trained muscles of stable patients with COPD. Function of the accessory inspiratory muscles and diaphragm show also important changes after training. Inspiratory muscle function can improve with specific training. It appears that there are significant gains after inspiratory muscle training and when intensity is monitored and exceeds 20% of maximal inspiratory pressure (PI $_{max}$). In this chapter, the extent to which muscle dysfunction can be improved, and the strategies by which to do so, are discussed.

Skeletal muscle function in COPD

Muscle function is distinguished largely by endurance and strength. Endurance is defined as the capacity of the muscle to maintain certain force overtime and strength is defined as the capacity of the muscle to develop maximal force to resist fatigue, loss of either one of these aspects results in skeletal muscle dysfunction and impaired skeletal muscle function thus, to resist fatigue. Loss of either one of these aspects results in muscle weakness and impaired muscle performance. Numerous studies have now convincingly shown that COPD is commonly associated with muscle weakness. However, strength and endurance seem not to be affected in the same way in respiratory and peripheral muscles. This is illustrated by the poor correlation between the strengths of both muscle groups in the 2 disorders compared with the much stronger correlation in healthy subjects. This implies that the strength component of muscle weakness is affected differently in peripheral and respiratory muscles. In healthy subjects as well as in patients with COPD, exercise-limiting symptoms are the sense of leg effort (exertional discomfort) or breathlessness (exertional dyspnea). Thus, despite correlations between peripheral muscle strength and performance in COPD, reduced endurance (ie, fatigue) seems to be the dominant limiting factor in peripheral muscles in these patients because the sense of leg effort was one of the main reasons to stop exercising.

It was shown that early lactic acidosis occurs in COPD during exercise and that this is largely the result of lactate release from the lower exercising limbs. Muscle acidosis is a contributing factor to muscle fatigue. Fatigue is probably not the main limiting factor in respiratory muscle function. Morrison et al found that COPD patients have low respiratory muscle strength and endurance. Fatigue of the respiratory muscles may indeed occur during exercise, but it is not certain whether this is an independent determinant of exercise capacity. In addition, it is unlikely that the respiratory muscles of exercising COPD patients contribute to the lactate response mentioned earlier. It should also be emphasized that the respiratory muscles must operate against the mechanical airway impedances in this specific disorder, for which the force component of respiratory muscle function is most likely of great importance.

Skeletal muscle dysfunction is very common in patients with COPD and may play an important role in limiting exercise performance in these patients. Muscle atrophy is largely responsible for the reduction in muscle strength. Changes in reduced capillarity, fiber type, decreased oxidative enzyme capacity, and altered cellular bioenergetics have all been documented in patients with COPD and can potentially explain the reduction in muscle endurance. Other systemic inflammatory such as malnutrition depletion, hypoxemia, disuse, Oxidative stress and medication may contribute to the observed muscle abnormalities that affect skeletal muscle function in COPD patients.

COPD is usually accompanied with extra-pulmonary abnormalities which are shown by a number of studies and it is called systemic effects of the disease. Abnormalities of skeletal muscle function and structure consider one of the best characterized systemic impacts of COPD which cause both skeletal muscle wasting and muscle dysfunction.

The diaphragm, the scalenus, and the parasternal intercostals consider primary muscles of inspiration and required within quiet breathing. The diaphragm achieves over 70% to 80% of the work of breathing, under quiet breathing conditions. Contraction of the diaphragm leads to the dome descends to compress the abdominal contents, shorten, and increasing intra-abdominal pressure that causes the lower rib cage to expand and decrease in intrathoracic pressure responsible for inspiration.Thus ,after facilitating an increase in pressure in the abdominal compartment instead of outward protrusion of the abdomen within contraction of the diaphragm.

During inspiration, the upward and outward rib move and based on the cranial orientation of the diaphragm's insertion. However, COPD patients may be caused by flattened of the diaphragm dome because the diaphragm fibers pull horizontally on the ribs instead of outward and upward. The scalene muscle arise on the lower five cervical vertebrae of the transverse processes and insert on the upper surface on the first and second ribs. Another important inspiratory muscle is the parasternal muscles that run among the castal cartilages in an outward and downward direction.The anterior-posterior dimension of the rib cage increases and the ribs are arisen when the parasternal muscles contract.

The expiratory action of the diaphragm on the upper rib cage is contracted by the inspiratory action of the scalene and parasternal muscle groups on the upper thorax. In addition, inspiration muscles have the most important accessory, it is called the sternocleidomastoid muscles which run from the mastoid processes to insert the medial third of the ventral surface of the manubrium stemi and clavicle. During inspiration, the sternocleidomastoid muscles contract when excess of the ventilator demands to increase the anteroposterior diameter of the upper rib cage and lift the sternum.

Muscular atrophy

Skeletal muscular atrophy is considered to be a significant feature of. Atrophy of the muscles means a reduction in fiber cross-sectional. Many agents influence the loss in fat-free mass (FFM) and body weight in patients with COPD. These agents include pulmonary inflammation, tissue hypoxia and an imbalance in overall protein turnover along with the hormones involved in this process. In addition there are some markers which correlate the atrophy that happens in patients with COPD to both oxidative stress-mediated and oxidative stress processes, for example atrophy, disruption of the excitation–contraction coupling, apoptosis and inflammation.

Muscle weight accounts for approximately 60-80% of fat-free mass FFM, so it can be used as evidence for muscle mass. Studies have shown that COPD patients lose their muscle mass especially in the lower limbs and upper limbs, thus complain of fatigue, dyspnoea and lose exercise endurance with just a minimal degree of exertion. This wastage compromises their ability to exercise, their cardiac fitness suffers and their exercise tolerance is limited, this then creates a vicious downward spiral which in the end results in immobility and generalized fatigue.

Several studies have found that there are ways to measure atrophy levels utilizing the plentiful markers in muscle extracts and incubated cells taken from muscles. There is an increase of proteolysis in many types of muscle atrophy, for example in the ATP dependent ubiquitin-proteasome pathway. In addition, many different muscle types display signs of atrophy relative to adaptations of the ubiquitin-proteasome pathway.

Fiber types

There are three fiber types in skeletal muscles; Type 1, Type 2A, and Type 2B, each type being identified by the isoform of myosin heavy chain. Type 1 fibers are resistant to fatigue, and are slow-twitch fibers with increased oxidative metabolism and they develop relatively small tension. Type 2A fibers are more general purpose and intermediate fatigue resistance. Type 2B fibers are highly susceptible to fatigue, fast-twitch fibers, based primarily on anaerobic glycolytic metabolism and develop high tension rates. However, the change in the ratio of fibers helps to maintain strength but at the cost of reduced muscle endurance and increased fatigability.

Intercostals muscles consist of a higher proportion of fast fibres, while human diaphragm contains equal proportions of the Fast fibers and slow fibers. A high aerobic oxidative enzyme activity, abundance of capillaries and a small fiber size are typical features of diaphragm fibers and give them the resistance to fatigue required by their continuous activity. Because of their fiber intercostals, composition muscles are less resistant to fatigue. The functional and structural characteristics of respiratory muscle fibres response to several pathological and physiological conditions such as training (adaptation to changes in respiratory load), age related changes, adaptation to hypoxia and changes associated with respiratory diseases. The properties of respiratory muscle fibers can also be modified by pharmacological agents such as b2 agonists and corticosteroids used for the treatment of respiratory diseases.

In COPD patients biopsies of the quadriceps muscle a reduction ratio of myosin heavy chain (MHC) type 1 fiber as compared with healthy controls (24.6 ± 7.1 versus 30.6 ± 6.7% ; P= 0.114), but there were no differences in the ratio of MHC type 2A fiber among patients and healthy controls. While, the ratio of MHC type 2B fibers increased in patients as compared with healthy controls (30.4 ± 5.7 versus 19.4 ± 10.9% ; P= 0.044).

There may be a decreasing ratio of fibers resulting from changes in the activation of the apoptotic pathways or in the regulation of skeletal muscle regeneration in COPD patients.

Actin-myosin isoforms

Fiber architecture is one of the unique features in skeletal muscle and is responsible for the functional capabilities of skeletal muscle due to the contribution of the highly organized arrangement of muscle fibers. The myosin molecule is composed of two heavy (MyHC) and two light chains (MyLC) that together with the adenosine triphosphatase (ATPase) activity, determine the functional characteristics of the fiber. Myosin is the most fundamental portion of the contractile machinery in muscle, and is found in many isoforms that contribute to the functional variety of muscle fibers. There are diverse functional types of myosin isoforms that form part of the heavy chain of the myosin molecule.

Myosin is a hexametric protein consisting of light and heavy chains which are essential for muscle contraction Figure (21).

COPD patients display changes in their skeletal muscle structure and function such as a reduction of contractile strength, a decrease of exercise tolerance and evidence of damage in their oxidative and energetic metabolism. There is also an alteration of fiber-type composition, with a reduction in the ratio of fatigue-resistant slow fibers.

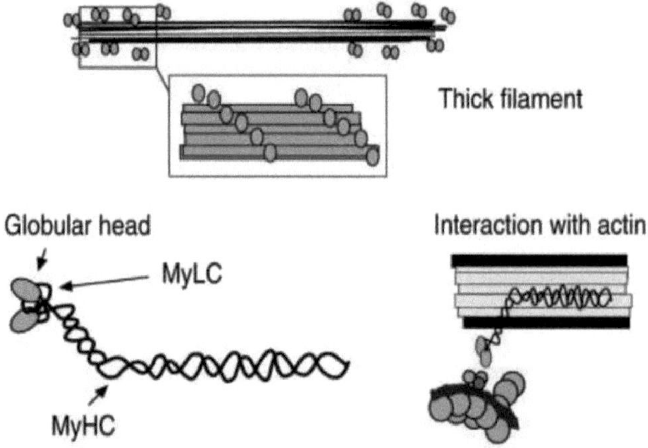

Fig 21. Molecular structure of myosin. MyLC: myosin light chain; MyHC: myosin heavy chain (Gea, 1997).

Biopsy specimens from the quadriceps femoris of COPD patients has been analyzed and has shown significant fiber wasting with a decreasing ratio of slow fibers and an associated increase in fast 2B fibers.

In the vastus lateralis of patients with COPD there was a noticeably increased expression of fast MyoLC and MyoHC 2B isoforms. COPD patients have lower percentage of fast MyoHC 2A and MyoHC 2B and a higher percentage of slow MyoHC than controls subjects. In addition, the diaphragm of COPD patients contain higher levels of tropomyosin and troponins, there is also a lower percentage of the slow isoforms of MyoLC than is evident in the control groups.

Respiratory muscle strength and endurance

Respiratory muscle in COPD patients is often weak and shows a decrease of endurance. There are many elements related to both the severity and presence of COPD that damage respiratory muscle structure and function. In addition, respiratory muscle in COPD patients bears a relationship with some important and relevant discoveries about differences in structure and function.

Many patients with COPD have impaired respiratory muscle function which has a significant adverse effect on their lives. Respiratory muscle is often weak and shows a decrease of endurance and strength because of the damaging that occurs in respiratory muscle structure and function, poor nutrition and hyperinflation. In addition, shorter operating lengths and higher speeds of shortening of the respiratory muscles during exercise and other daily activities which require high ventilation levels.

The differences between normal individuals and COPD patients in respiratory muscle strength and endurance were less in COPD patients compared with normal subjects. Respiratory muscle endurance in patients with COPD is compromised more than respiratory muscle strength.

Respiratory muscle endurance and strength training in COPD

Patients with COPD have a decrease in respiratory muscle endurance and strength because of poor nutrition, hyperinflation and general condition. Respiratory muscle endurance training can be defined as: " *repetitive shortening contractions that are in coordination with the breathing pattern* ". Whereas, respiratory muscle strength training can be defined as: " *the performance of high, near-maximal inspiratory or expiratory maneuvers that are usually quasi-isometric*".

Several studies have investigated the role of respiratory muscle training in COPD patients that have aimed to improve respiratory muscle endurance rather than respiratory muscle strength. Such studies have typically reported only insignificant improvements in dyspnoea scores, exercise tolerance and quality of life. Smith *et al.* (1992) found little evidence of clinically important benefits of IMT beyond an improvement in results of respiratory muscle endurance tests. Although randomized controlled trials that evaluated the effect of respiratory muscle training were considered, no distinction was made between trials of IMT vs conventional care and trials in which IMT was added to exercise therapy. In addition, Mador *et al.* (2005) found that respiratory muscle endurance training does not improve in quality of life or exercise performance. In contrast, Scherer *et al.* (2000) found that respiratory muscle endurance training with normocapnichyperpnea improves dyspnoea, health-related quality of life, exercise performance and respiratory muscle in COPD patients. Therefore, the findings of Sturdy *et al.* (2003) reported that respiratory muscle endurance training increase PI_{max} 32 ± 27% in COPD patients because of improving respiratory neuromuscular coordination.

Very little researches into the effects of respiratory muscle strength training have been conducted in COPD patients. When comparing the relative merits of strength versus endurance training. Respiratory muscle strength training uses to improve muscle strength and maximal sustainable ventilation capacity or maximal voluntary ventilation.

When added strength training to an endurance exercise program can produce significant improvements in muscle strength in patients with COPD.

Recently studies have used threshold loading, maximal sustained voluntary ventilation and inspiratory resistive breathing techniques to improve the respiratory muscle endurance and strength training and then quality of life in patients with COPD. The result studies were different, Reid and Samrai (1995) using targeted inspiratory resistive and threshold training to improve respiratory muscles in COPD patients. In addition, Goldstein *et al.* (1989) showed that training using threshold loading improves significantly inspiratory muscle endurance but not muscle strength. In contrast, Weiner and colleagues (1992) found that training for 6 months by using threshold loading improves inspiratory muscle endurance and strength.

To my personal knowledge, the different results for these studies to improve dyspnoea and quality of life by using respiratory muscle endurance and strength training are due to small attention to training intensity, study design, outcome measures and statistical power that will help to provide better guidance regarding the role of respiratory muscle training in pulmonary rehabilitation programs.

Upper torso and arm training

Exercise training for patients with chronic obstructive pulmonary disease (COPD) has traditionally emphasized lower-extremity exercise (eg, walking, cycling); however, many patients with COPD report disabling dyspnoea for daily activities involving the upper extremities (eg, brushing teeth, bathing) at work levels much lower than for lower-extremity exercise.

Upper limb muscles training programs are important to improve the quality of life and decreased the dyspnoea in COPD patients. These programs result in significant changes on isotonic arm cycle, simulated activities of daily-living and ventilatory muscle endurance tests in patients with severe COPD. In addition, arm training can increase ability to perform unsupported arm exercise and improve endurance and strength of upper muscles in subjects with COPD. Moreover, specific training programs for the arms may lead to a decrease in dyspnoea and an improvement in the quality of life for COPD patients.

Relatively few studies examine the use of upper-limb exercise training for patients with COPD. The studies evaluating the rationale for and outcomes of arm training for COPD patients have been reviewed elsewhere. In brief, arm training has been studied because patients with moderate to severe COPD, particularly those with mechanical disadvantage of the diaphragm due to lung hyperinflation, have difficulty performing ADLs that involve the use of the upper limbs. Also, arm elevation is associated with high metabolic and ventilatory demand, and activities involving the arms can lead to irregular, shallow, or dyssynchronous breathing. An altered breathing pattern may result from de-recruitment of accessory respiratory muscles from their work as muscles of inspiration to contribute to arm activity. Upper-limb exercise may cause a shift in the load of breathing to the mechanically disadvantaged diaphragm, with resultant ventilatory limitation during arm activities. Although skeletal muscle dysfunction plays a significant role in exercise limitation of the lower limb, the dyspnea experienced during arm exercise is likely more related to the above-noted patterns of muscle use, and is less likely primarily dependent on inherent skeletal muscle dysfunction of the upperlimb. Indeed, studies of the anatomical and physiologic derangements of skeletal muscle in COPD have demonstrated that upper-limb muscles are affected to a lesser degree than lower-limb muscles. This is likely due to the patient's tendency to eliminate first those activities that involve the muscles of ambulation, leading to overall deconditioning. In contrast, arm activities are still required for maintenance of self-care and independent living, even if they induce uncomfortable symptoms of dyspnea and fatigue. Nevertheless, improvements in upper-limb strength or endurance resulting from training could lead to improved overall functional capacity and ability to perform ADLs.

Upper-limb muscle training may consist of endurance training (via arm ergometry [supported exercise], or unsupported, arm-lifting exercise), or strength training (weight lifting. Reported benefits of upper-limb training in COPD include improved arm muscle endurance and strength, reduced metabolic demand associated with arm exercise, and improved sense of well-being. In general, benefits of upper-limb training are task-specific; that is, improvements are noted only in performance of the types of tasks for which the muscle groups were trained. Since upper-limb training is generally safe, does not necessarily require use of specialized equipment, and is easily incorporated into most exercise programs, the AACVPR/ACCP Joint Evidence-Based Guidelines Panel and the ATS Statement on Pulmonary Rehabilitation recommend that upper limb training be included routinely as a component of the rehabilitation of patients with COPD. Further study is needed to determine whether routine use of arm training, particularly when combined with lower-limb training, can lead to consistent improvements in overall endurance and the ability to perform ADLs.

Exercise Tolerance and Quality of Life

COPD is a progressive disorder and the worsening dyspnoea and ongoing loss of exercise tolerance progressively impairs the COPD patient's quality of life. By the time that the FEV_1 has fallen to below 30% of the predicted levels, COPD patients are normally breathless on minimal exertion. Various exercise tests are therefore widely used to evaluate exercise tolerance in COPD patients. Free walking tests such as the 6 minute walk test, constant work rate test, and incremental exercise tests are used in COPD patients to assess exercise tolerance and to evaluate improvement of exercise tolerance from therapeutic interventions such as pulmonary rehabilitation programs.

Quality of life can be assessed by questionnaire instruments such as the Chronic Respiratory Questionnaire (CRQ) which examines four dimensions: mastery, fatigue, emotion, and dyspnoea. Such instruments are useful in COPD patients for evaluating the effects on quality of life of inspiratory muscle training and exercise training. Other QoL instruments were designed to provide a standardized method by which health status or levels of health impairment could be measured and compared in individual patients as well as in groups of patients. HRQL instruments included: St George's Respiratory Questionnaire (SGRQ), Sickness Impact Profile (SIP), Hospital Anxiety and Depression Scale and Mood Adjective Check List.

Type and intensity of training

The optimal type and intensity of training for patients with COPD remains the subject of debate. While all types of training can improve exercise performance, different outcomes can be expected depending on whether the patient undertakes aerobic endurance versus strength training, whether high- or low-intensity training is chosen, and whether upper-limb and/or respiratory muscle training is pursued in addition to lower-limb training. No single exercise formula can be considered ideal for all persons. The exercise program must be individually tailored to meet the needs and goals of the patient, using resources available.

Aerobic Versus Strength Training

In general, aerobic fitness (endurance) training improves one's ability to sustain an exercise task at a given work load. Walking, running, cycling, stair climbing and swimming are examples of endurance training exercise. In contrast, strength training involves bursts of activity over a shorter period, such as occur during weight lifting. Each of these forms of training can be undertaken at high or low intensity; that is, at high or low percentages of the patient's individual maximal work capacity for the given task. Many clinical trials of exercise training in COPD, such as the study by Ries and colleagues, have used aerobic endurance exercise such as cycling as the principal or sole mode of exercise training.

As reviewed above, lower-limb aerobic fitness training leads to gains in exercise endurance, and to a lesser degree, gains in maximal work load. Fewer studies have evaluated the impact of strength training as a sole exercise modality for persons with COPD. Resistance training improves leg strength and walking distance in healthy elderly persons. Simpson and colleagues demonstrated a 73 percent increase in cycling endurance time at 80 percent of maximal power output following 8 weeks of weight lifting training of the upper- and lowerlimb muscles of patients with COPD. Of note, there was no concomitant improvement in 6 MWD. In another study, weight training of the upper and lower limbs led to improved muscle function and treadmill walking endurance in patients with mild COPD who had impaired isokinetic lower-limb muscle function prior to training [126],

and the noted improvements in muscle strength correlated with improvements in muscle endurance. The relative advantages and disadvantages of high- versus lowintensity strength training for persons with COPD are as yet unknown. Safety, especially prevention of muscle

tears, is of paramount importance, particularly for persons on chronic steroid treatment who may be at risk for muscle rupture (e.g., biceps) when exposed to a high-intensity load. Clearly, such rupture can lead to prolonged, if not permanent, additional functional disability. A recommended approach for strength training prescription has been reviewed recently. Since both aerobic fitness/endurance training and weight training can be beneficial and are safe for patients with COPD (when administered properly), most rehabilitation programs currently use both types of training. The best way to combine these training strategies is, however, still unclear. Spruit and colleagues compared the effects of dynamic strength exercise to those of endurance training (walking, cycling, and arm cranking) during a 12-week rehabilitation program in 48 patients with severe COPD.

Significant improvements in muscle force and torque, 6 MWD, Wmax, and health-related QOL were noted for patients in both groups, and the two training types led to a similar magnitude of gains. However, the substantial intersubjective variability raised questions as to whether some subjects may have derived benefit more from one versus the other form of training. Bernard and colleagues conducted a randomized trial of 12 weeks of aerobic endurance training, alone or in combination with strength training, in 36 patients with moderate to severe COPD. Whereas muscle strength increased to a greater degree in the combined training group, the addition of strength training to aerobic endurance training did not lead to greater improvements in peak work rate, 6 MWD, or QOL assessed by the CRQ. More recently, Ortega and colleagues also compared the effects of 12 weeks of strength training, endurance training, or a combination approach in 47 patients with COPD.

Greater improvements in submaximal exercise capacity were noted among persons who had endurance training as part of their regimen, and greater improvements in muscle strength were found in subjects whose regimen included strength training. Overall, similarly to the study by Bernard [68], there was no clear noted additive or synergistic effect of combination therapy on exercise performance as compared with either modality alone, and the training effects were consistent with the type(s) of training undertaken. Although to date there exist no clear proven benefits of combined modality training, there likely are subgroups of individuals that might benefit particularly from this approach. Also, the ability to perform day-to-day activities may be a more important outcome to detect beneficial effects, as compared to a limited profile of program-based, standardized strength and endurance tests. However, as noted, a limited number of tools exist to accurately assess and quantitatively measure ADL performance. Thus, since both interventions are generally safe, it is reasonable to include both aerobic and strength training in the exercise program of most persons with COPD.

High- Versus Low-Intensity Aerobic Fitness (Endurance) Training

Assessment of Exercise Intensity: Identification of Target Work Load

In general, high-intensity exercise is considered to be that which takes place at greater than 60 percent of the patient's VO2max or Wmax, whereas lower intensity exercise is conducted at lower work rates. Historically, several methods have been used to define the exercise intensity used in clinical trials of exercise training in COPD. The use of target heart rate (HR) may not be a reliable indicator of consistently chosen target work rate in this patient population. The HR at estimated lactate threshold varies as a percentage of predicted peak HR, and percentage of heart rate reserve (HRR), and a specific HR achieved during training may correlate to variable work rates, depending on the severity and stability of the cardiopulmonary disease over time. Cardiopulmonary exercise testing (CPET), wherein the work rate is measured directly, is the most direct means of assessing exercise intensity. However, comprehensive CPET is not mandated in all patients prior to PR, and it is not available at all centers. The incremental SWT is an acceptable noninvasive alternate field test that can be used to guide training intensity. Performance in this test correlates well to VO2max measured during an incremental CPET. Thus, a specific target training work load can be derived from the maximal speed achieved during the SWT. Persons with very advanced disease and severe functional impairment who are unable to perform standardized walk tests or CPET can be exercised to the tolerable limits of dyspnea and/or leg fatigue.

Assessment of Physiologic Changes Following Training

A separate issue is how to measure whether physiologic changes associated with improved aerobic fitness have occurred following training. CPET is the standard means of measuring VO2max, Wmax, and lactate threshold, and of comparing values before and after exercise

training [133]. Muscle biopsies can be used to detect structural and metabolic changes following training, but are usually conducted for this purpose only in a research setting. More recently, it has been appreciated that biomarkers such as exhaled nitric oxide (NO) may be of use in assessing the physiologic response to exercise training. Exhaled NO has been identified as a marker of physical fitness in healthy subjects [134]. Increases in exhaled NO have also been associated with improvements in exercise tolerance following PR for persons with COPD. The routine clinical utility of this measure is as yet unknown.

Outcomes of High-Intensity Endurance Training

High-intensity exercise must be undertaken for the patient to gain significant physiologic improvements in aerobic fitness. Characteristic physiologic changes indicating improvements in aerobic fitness following exercise training include increased muscle fiber capillarization, mitochondrial density and oxidative capacity of muscle fibers, and delay of the onset of anaerobic metabolism during exercise (i.e., ability to exercise to a higher work rate before reaching the anaerobic/lactate threshold). These factors in turn lead to reduced ventilatory requirement for a given exercise task, increased VO2max and decreased HR for a given oxygen consumption (VO2). The demonstration of improvements in one or more of these variables following exercise training in patients with COPD is evidence of physiologic improvement in aerobic fitness. For many years, the efficacy of exercise training was questioned, since persons with severe FEV1 impairment were thought to be too ventilatory-limited to achieve gains in aerobic fitness [137]. Subsequent studies have shown convincingly, however, that many (although not all) patients with severely impaired lung function can tolerate moderate- to high-intensity endurance training and can achieve significant physiologic gains in aerobic fitness. For example, Casaburi compared the effects of cycle ergometry training (45 min/ day for 8 weeks) at a high-intensity work load (mean 71W) to those following training at a low-intensity work load (mean 30 W) in 19 patients with moderate COPD (FEV1 56 ± 12% predicted). Training led to reductions in lactate production and VE requirement for identical work rates in both groups, but the magnitude of physiologic improvement was much greater in the subjects trained at the high work rate. Also, cycle endurance time increased by 73 percent in the high-intensity group, and by only 9 percent in the low-intensity group. Maltais *et al.* also demonstrated physiologic gains in aerobic fitness following 12 weeks of exercise training (30 min/day,

3 days/ week) at a work rate corresponding to 80 percent of the VO2max in persons with severe COPD (FEV1 36 ± 11% predicted) [44]. Similar improvements in physiologic parameters of aerobic fitness following high- but not low intensity endurance training have been confirmed in several additional studies. Importantly, whereas moderate- to high-intensity exercise is needed to make gains in aerobic fitness, it is not always necessary that the exercise intensity be so high that the patient reaches anaerobic threshold. Improvements in VO2max and maximal treadmill work load and reduced symptoms of dyspnea and fatigue can occur following moderate- to high-intensity exercise, even among persons who do not reach anaerobic threshold. Moreover, not all patients can tolerate high-intensity exercise at the outset of training. It likely is important, however, that such patients exercise to the maximum intensity tolerated to achieve gains in aerobic fitness. Those who do can achieve gains in the maximum intensity of exercise tolerated over time. This was demonstrated by Maltais and colleagues, who evaluated 42 patients with severe COPD (mean FEV1 38 ± 13% predicted) at baseline and after 12 weeks of cycle ergometer endurance training. Although the intended target training intensity was 80 percent of Wmax, the actual average tolerated training intensity by week 2 was only 24.5 ± 12.6 percent Wmax for this group of patients. However, by week 12, the same patients were able to exercise, on average, at 60 ± 22.7 percent of Wmax. Patients not only achieved significant increases in Wmax from training, but also made significant improvements in VO2max and had reductions in VE and arterial lactate concentration for exercise at a given
work rate following training.

Interval training (alternating periods of high- vs. low intensity exercise or rest) is another option for persons who cannot sustain extended, continuous periods of high intensity exercise. Two recent studies have confirmed the efficacy of interval training in improving exercise tolerance. Importantly, interval exercise more closely resembles the type of exercise output required for ADLs than does continuous high-intensity exercise.

The physiologic response to interval training depends on the precise structure, i.e., nature and intensity, of the program, and on the study population chosen. Physiologic gains in aerobic fitness can occur.

Moderate- to high-intensity training likely leads to improved aerobic fitness, at least in part by enhancing the activity of skeletal muscle oxidative enzymes. Maltais and colleagues found reduced activity of the oxidative enzymes citrate synthase and 3-hydroxyacyl Co A dehydrogenase before training in 11 persons with severe COPD. The activity of these enzymes increased significantly after high-intensity exercise training, and the noted improvement correlated to the reduction in lactic acid during exercise. Moreover, reductions in ventilator requirement following training are associated with increased Vt and lower respiratory rate, with a resultant decrease in Vd/Vt.

Reduction in the activity of the proteolytic proteasome pathway of metabolism is another mechanism by which physical training may lead to improved muscle function. It is important to consider whether any detrimental effects of high-intensity training exist for persons with COPD. A few studies have addressed this issue. To determine if high-intensity exercise leads to diaphragmatic fatigue, twitch diaphragmatic pressure was measured during cervical magnetic stimulation before and at sequential intervals after high-intensity cycling exercise (to the time of intolerable symptoms) in 12 patients with moderate to severe COPD. Of the 12 subjects, only two developed evidence of contractile diaphragmatic fatigue, whereas the majority of patients tolerated high intensity exercise without adverse effect. However, in a different type of study, Orozco-Levi found that the diaphragm muscle in patients with COPD may be susceptible to sarcomere disruption, and this effect can be

exacerbated by threshold inspiratory loading. It is not clear whether such injury could be induced by high intensity exercise. Quadriceps fatigue has been reported following high-intensity exercise. One further study cautions that, although endurance exercise improves muscle redox potential in healthy persons, moderate intensity training can lead to reduced muscle redox capacity in patients with severe COPD. Such an

effect could potentially lead to worsened, rather than improved, skeletal muscle function in some patients, by virtue of exaggerating oxidative stress. Further work is needed to clarify which patients are at greatest risk for this potentially detrimental training effect, and which are likely to improve oxidative enzyme capacity following training. Identification of persons who may be at risk of diaphragm fatigue and exaggerated oxidative stress or other detrimental training effects, and an understanding of the impact of these effects on exercise tolerance and functional status long-term, would be useful in designing optimal exercise strategies for individuals. Finally, it must be noted that improvement in the physiologic parameters of aerobic fitness following high intensity exercise is not absolutely necessary to achieve improvements in exercise tolerance. This is important, since......

(1) high-intensity exercise may lead to a greater degree of dyspnea/leg fatigue and may therefore be less likely to be incorporated into the patient's routine lifestyle;

(2) some persons cannot tolerate high-intensity exercise, and

(3) as noted, some may develop deleterious muscle effects. Moreover, it has not been proven conclusively that aerobic fitness (with such physiologic gains as increased VO2max and decreased lactate, VE, etc.) results in better improvement in day-to-day functional capacity than lower intensity exercise (which does not lead to these physiologic training effects).

Outcomes of Low-Intensity Training

It has been demonstrated clearly that lower intensity exercise also leads to improved exercise tolerance, even in the absence of measured physiologic gains in aerobic fitness. For example, striking gains in treadmill endurance without increases in VO2max were noted in the randomized-controlled trial of outpatient PR conducted by Ries et al. as well as in another study evaluating the effects of low-intensity isolated peripheral muscle exercise in 48 patients with severe COPD.

Low intensity multimodality exercise training also led to increased exercise tolerance for patients undergoing inpatient PR. Gains in endurance and/or strength may be seen following such low-intensity exercise training. Two recent studies have directly compared the clinical benefits of high- versus low-intensity exercise training. In these trials, gains in exercise endurance were noted following both types of training, although the magnitude of gain was greater among the patients who had higher intensity exercise. However, the study by Normandin, found that the low-intensity training group had greater increases in arm endurance, and both groups achieved comparable reductions in overall dyspnea, functional performance, and health status. Recently, two studies have reported the effects of transcutaneous neuromuscular electrical stimulation (NMES) on the exercise tolerance of patients with COPD. In one, improvements in muscle strength and endurance, whole body exercise endurance, and dyspnea were noted following NMES. Compliance with the regimen was excellent and, notably, subjects were able to continue the training regimen despite the occurrence of intermittent disease exacerbations. Similarly, Bourjeily- Habr and colleagues demonstrated that transcutaneous electrical stimulation of the lower-limb muscle led to improved quadriceps and hamstring muscle strength with associated improvements in distance completed in the SWT. Importantly, in both of these studies, the noted benefits were achieved even without conventional concomitant strength or endurance training. Transcutaneous electrical muscle stimulation may be particularly beneficial for patients with very severe disease who are unable or unwilling to participate in a conventional exercise training program.

The mechanisms by which exercise tolerance/endurance improves following low-intensity exercise, wherein no specific improvements in aerobic fitness are noted, are not fully elucidated. However, gains in peripheral or respiratory muscle strength, increased mechanical efficiency of performing exercise due to improved neuromuscular coupling and coordination, reduction in hyperinflation/
improved lung emptying, reduced anxiety and dyspnea, and improved motivation may all play a role. Different combinations of mechanisms likely result in the improvements noted in individual persons.

Exercise-induced respiratory muscle fatigue

The structural and functional properties of the respiratory muscles appear to be well suited to the ventilatory requirements of exercise. For example, the human at rest can sustain up to six to eight times the resting diaphragmatic pressure production for 10 to 15 minutes without inducing significant fatigue or task failure of the diaphragm. Furthermore, pressures and velocities of shortening sustained by the diaphragm which is 1.5 to 2 times greater than those attained during exhaustive exercise are required to cause diaphragm fatigue when the subject is in the resting state and increases ventilation voluntarily. Nevertheless, significant 15 to 50% reductions in the transdiaphragmatic pressure response to bilateral phrenic nerve stimulation, across a wide range of stimulation frequencies (1 to 100Hz) and lung volumes residual volume to TLC, have been observed following constant-load, whole body endurance exercise. The magnitude of exercise-induced diaphragm fatigue is determined in part by the amount of diaphragm work contributing to the exercise hyperpnea. Thus, reducing the pressures produced by the diaphragm during endurance exercise with the use of a proportional assist ventilator prevented diaphragm fatigue.80 Popular predictors of fatigue, such as the pressure–time index of the diaphragm and the ratio of transdiaphragmatic pressure to maximal transdiaphragmatic pressure, were unable to show consistently whether the diaphragmatic force output during exercise was sufficient to cause diaphragm fatigue. Indeed, exercise-induced diaphragm fatigue occurred most often when the values of these indices were only one-half to two-thirds those required to produce fatigue under resting conditions. Thus, although these indices are adequate predictors of task failure during sustained voluntary efforts against an inspiratory resistive load in resting subjects, they are not during whole body exercise. Whole body exercise

itself appears to lower the threshold of force output by the diaphragm required for its fatigue, probably because a finite blood flow must be distributed to both locomotor and respiratory muscles. Such a disparity between oxygen supply and demand appears to occur in subjects of varying fitness levels, but only at workloads exceeding 85% of ˙VO2MAX or when arterial oxygen content is decreased.

Effect of exercise training on the lower extremities

Results from a meta-analysis of randomized trials with comparable patient selection and training modalities conducted over the last 40 years clearly show that pulmonary rehabilitation improves the functional capacity and the health related quality of life of patients with COPD. In addition to an educational component, rehabilitation programs generally include a component that focuses on breathing strategies to minimize breathlessness and optimize breathing mechanics in addition to a large muscle mass exercise training component. The exercise training programs have typically been structured around supervised institutional programs ranging from 4 weeks up to 1 year in duration (mode: 8 weeks) consisting of treadmill walking, stationary cycling, and free-walking. Over the last decade, strength training of either lower or upper extremities has also been introduced as a valuable adjunctive exercise rehabilitation modality in patients with COPD. Similarly, an increasing number of studies have addressed the long-term effectiveness of home-based exercise training on functional status, quality of life, and the long-term adherence to physical activity training. Outcome measures of the effectiveness of the exercise training programs on functional or physical performance indicators have been obtained from direct open circuit spirometer measurements during incremental maximal exercise tests but more often from exercise tests using a fixed absolute submaximal power output or using a timed-distance field test. Most studies have assessed subjects with mild or moderate disease severity; however, improvements in exercise tolerance have also been observed in

severely impaired patients.

Effects of weight training

Peripheral muscle strength is considerably reduced in patients with COPD, and irrespective of lung function, impairment is negatively related to overall exercise capacity. It therefore seems reasonable that weight training be recommended in patients in COPD. Nonetheless, there are, to date, a relatively small number of randomized trials of weight lifting in COPD. Most trials have used a training modality consisting of three series of 10 movement repetitions of low or moderate intensity with respect to the maximal strength of the target muscle group, including both lower and upper limb muscle masses. Similar to healthy individuals, significant gains in the strength of the exercised muscle groups may be observed following strength training, indicating that the disease process does not impair muscle tissue trainability in COPD. In fact, improvements in muscle endurance have also been reported following unloaded callisthenic-type exercises, which may be explained by the relatively weak baseline status. Although strength gains are specifically associated with strength rather than aerobic training, programs using combined strength and aerobic exercise training lead to improvements in strength of a magnitude similar to that of strength training alone. It is interesting that contrary to observations in healthy populations, increases in peripheral muscle strength transfer to improvements in submaximal endurance time and quality of life. This may be related to the fact that some patients with COPD are so low on the exercise fitness continuum that a small initial gain in peripheral muscle strength or endurance may make a difference to their ability to sustain longer bouts of physical activity using this muscle mass.

Weight training is associated with distinct advantages in patients with chronic diseases such as COPD, coronary heart disease, or congestive heart failure because the metabolic demands of segmental or localized muscle contractions and thus the related circulatory and ventilatory requirements remain significantly lower than for large muscle group exercise training. Patients can therefore perform substantial exercise without experiencing adverse symptoms such as pain or breathlessness.

Circuit training is a training modality that combines both weight lifting and aerobic training as subjects successively move two or three times through a circuit consisting of 6 to 10 stations and performing series of 10 to 12 repetitions of a given exercise at each weight lifting station using several upper and lower limb muscle groups. This approach has been used safely and successfully in cardiac rehabilitation programs, resulting in significant increases in both aerobic endurance and musculoskeletal strength. The use of this training modality in patients with COPD is restricted to series of consecutive arm exercises in upper extremity training but otherwise remains relatively unexplored.

Effect of exercise training on the upper extremities

The oxygen cost per $kg \cdot min\_1$ of arm ergometry is higher during arm cycling ($3mL \cdot kg\_1 \cdot min\_1$) compared with leg cycling ($2mL \cdot kg\_1 \cdot min\_1$) on account of the additional involvement of upper body stabilizing muscles during arm exercise. In addition, in untrained individuals, the maximal work capacity achieved using arm ergometry is approximately 64 to 80% of that achieved using lower extremities. Thus, for a given absolute work rate, the relative demands when performed with the upper limb muscles are much greater, leading to greater cardiorespiratory responses. Given

these factors, it is difficult to determine the appropriate grounds for comparison of arm and leg exercise responses following a given therapeutic intervention. In a recent study, investigators examined the efficiency of energy expenditure during peak and submaximal arm and leg cycling in patients with COPD.32 In agreement with the known effects of arm exercise, in the healthy control subjects, the VO2 per watt of peak external work was higher during arm (15.5 _ 0.7mL O2·min_1/W_1) than leg (10.0_ 0.3mL O2·min_1/W_1) ergometry. In patients, however, the VO2 per watt of peak external work was the same during arm (17.3_ 0.6 mL O2·min_1/W_1) and leg (17.3_ 0.7mL O2·min_1/W_1) ergometry. The mechanical efficiency (%), measured at an intensity of work corresponding to 50% of the specific arm or leg peak exercise performance, was significantly lower in patients than control subjects for legs (15.6_ 0.6 vs 22.5_0.6) but not for arm ergometry, for which a normal mechanical efficiency was observed (18.3_ 0.9 vs 21_ 1.2). This
suggests that upper and lower limbs are not comparably affected in COPD, although a clear explanation remains to be determined.

Evidence indicating that muscles of the upper limbs are equally affected by disuse or chronic hypoxemia was published by Sato and colleagues,33 showing type II fiber atrophy in the biceps muscle of patients with severe emphysema as is reported in the lower limb muscles of patients with COPD.21,34 On the other hand, recent results from biopsies of deltoid muscles in COPD patients indicate comparable and even higher oxidative enzyme activity than that of age-matched control subjects when only severe patients were considered. The deltoid muscle, however, is responsible for arm elevation and abduction, as well as fixation of the shoulder joint, but may also be recruited upon increased respiratory efforts. Similar to the recent report of a "supranormal" oxidative capacity of the costal diaphragm and external intercostal muscles of emphysematous patients,36 the higher citrate synthase activity observed in the deltoid muscle of severe COPD patients could be explained by an enhanced recruitment of the deltoid in light of the exaggerated work of breathing. Patients also report increased dyspnea when completing daily tasks involving arm movement, to displace objects or to raise arms above head level, referred to as "unsupported arm exercise," compared with leg exercise. The main problem in studying the physiologic responses to unsupported arm exercise and the potential related benefits of therapeutic interventions on responses to this exercise is the lack of standardization of the mechanical work and the resulting energy requirements. Because in unsupported arm exercise the amount of force displaced is not known, there cannot be a valid computation of the mechanical work. In addition, unsupported arm exercise involves the participation of accessory inspiratory muscles for stabilization of the torso to different degrees depending on the type of movement, which further complicates the bioenergetics assessment.

Upper extremity training using arm ergometry, weight lifting, or rhythmic unsupported arm movements using a wooden dowel have been successfully used in patients with COPD to improve dyspnea and arm working capacity. These studies show significant improvements in maximal arm work capacity or endurance following upper extremity training and support the principle of exercise-induced specificity of training since crossover effects of leg exercise training alone on arm exercise performance was not observed. Additional randomized controlled trials are required in these patients to further examine the added benefits of upper extremity training on functional ability, ventilator discomfort, and the resulting skeletal muscle metabolic or circulatory adaptations.

Chapter Five

Different Exercises for COPD Patients

With COPD, the less you do, the less you're able to do. Weak muscles need more oxygen, so you can become short of breath just shopping or cooking. Exercise changes that. When your muscles are stronger, daily activities are easier.

Every exercise session should include a **warm-up**, **conditioning phase**, and a **cool down**. The warm-up helps your body adjust slowly from rest to exercise.

A **warm-up** reduces the stress on your heart and muscles, slowly increases your breathing, circulation (heart rate), and body temperature. It also helps improve flexibility and reduce muscle soreness.

The best warm-up includes stretching, range of motion activities, and beginning of the activity at a low intensity level.

The **conditioning phase** follows the warm-up. During this phase, the benefits of exercise are gained and calories are burned. During the conditioning phase, you should monitor the intensity of the activity.

The intensity is how hard you are exercising, which can be measured by checking your heart rate. Your health care provider can give you more information on monitoring your heart rate.

Over time, you can work on increasing the duration of the activity. The duration is how long you exercise during one session.

The **cool-down** phase is the last phase of your exercise session. It allows your body to gradually recover from the conditioning phase. Your heart rate and blood pressure will return to near resting values. Cool-down does not mean to sit down. In fact, do not sit, stand still, or lie down right after exercise. This might cause you to feel dizzy, lightheaded, or have heart palpitations (fluttering in your chest).

The best cool-down is to slowly decrease the intensity of your activity. You might also do some of the same stretching activities you did in the warm-up phase.

General exercise guidelines:

- Gradually increase your activity level, especially if you have not been exercising regularly.
- Remember to have fun. Choose an activity you enjoy. Exercising should be fun and not a chore. You'll be more likely to stick with an exercise program if you enjoy the activity. Here are some questions you can think about before choosing a routine:
    - What physical activities do I enjoy?
    - Do I prefer group or individual activities?
    - What programs best fit my schedule?
    - Do I have physical conditions that limit my choice of exercise?
    - What goals do I have in mind? (losing weight, strengthening muscles, or improving flexibility, for example)
- Wait at least 1½ hours after eating a meal before exercising.
- When drinking liquids during exercise, remember to follow your fluid restriction guidelines.
- Dress for the weather conditions and wear protective footwear.
- Take time to include a five-minute warm-up, including stretching exercises, before any aerobic activity and include a five- to 10-minute cool down after the activity. Stretching can be done while standing or sitting.
- Schedule exercise into your daily routine. Plan to exercise at the same time every day (such as in the mornings when you have more energy). Add a variety of exercises so you do not get bored.
- Exercise at a steady pace. Keep a pace that allows you to still talk during the activity.

- Exercise does not have to put a strain on your wallet. Avoid buying expensive equipment or health club memberships unless you are certain you will use them regularly.
- Stick with it. If you exercise regularly, it will soon become part of your lifestyle. Make exercise a lifetime commitment. Finding an exercise "buddy" will also help you stay motivated.
- Keep an exercise record.

Breathing during activity:

Always breathe slowly to save your breath. Inhale through your nose, keeping your mouth closed. This warms and moisturizes the air you breathe and at the same time filters it. Exhale through pursed lips.

- Breathe out slowly and gently through pursed lips. This permits more complete lung action when the oxygen you inhale is exchanged for the carbon dioxide you exhale.
- Try to inhale for two seconds and exhale for four seconds. You might find slightly shorter or longer periods are more natural for you. If so, just try to breathe out twice as long as you breathe in.
- Exercise will not harm your lungs. When you experience shortness of breath during an activity, this is an indication that your body needs more oxygen. If you slow your rate of breathing and concentrate on exhaling through pursed lips, you will restore oxygen to your system more rapidly.

Some types of exercises:

1. Walk:

Just about everyone with COPD can exercise. Walking is a great choice, especially if you're just getting started. Do it anywhere -- outside, in a mall, on a treadmill. If it seems daunting, add 30 seconds or 10 yards each day. Even a slow pace will do you good. If you haven't been active lately, check with your doctor before starting an exercise program.

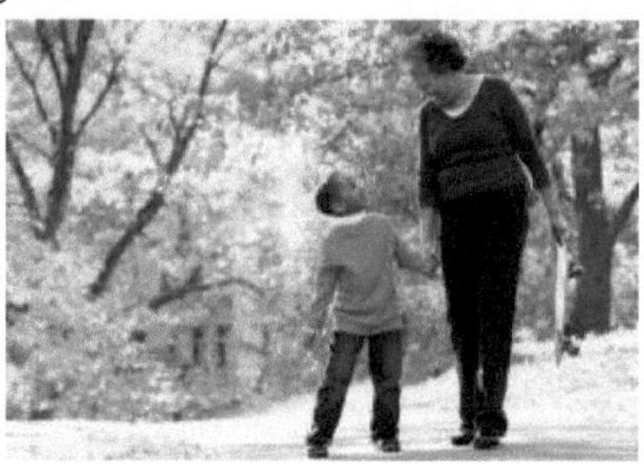

2. Bike:

A stationary bike can work well for people with COPD. You can pedal away in the privacy of your home. In a gym or rehab setting, you can find supervision and meet people. Ask the instructor before jumping into a group cycling class, to be sure it matches your ability. As you improve, try a spin outside on a traditional bike and soak up the scenery. If any exercise makes you short of breath, stop and sit down for a few minutes.

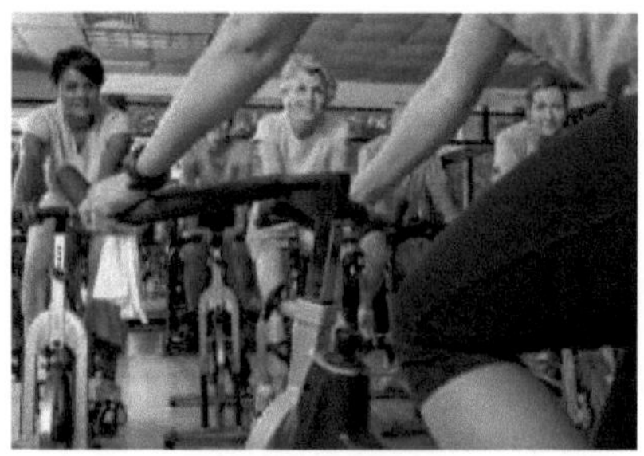

3. Arm Curls:

Lifting light weights can help you reach a high shelf or lug a gallon of milk. Choose hand weights, stretchy bands, or water bottles to try arm curls. Hold the weights at your sides, palms forward. Breathe in. Now lift toward your chest, keeping elbows down, and exhaling slowly. Slowly lower your arms back down as you breathe in. Build up to two sets of 10-15 repetitions.

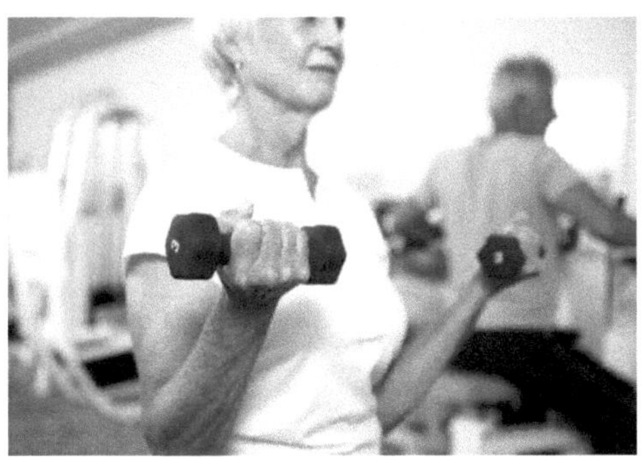

4. Forward Arm Raises:

Hold weights down at your sides, palms facing in. Inhale, then exhale slowly as you raise both arms straight out front to shoulder height. Inhale as you slowly lower your arms. This strengthens your upper arms and shoulders. Build up to two sets of 10-15 repetitions. Start with light weights and go a little heavier every two to three weeks to challenge your muscles.

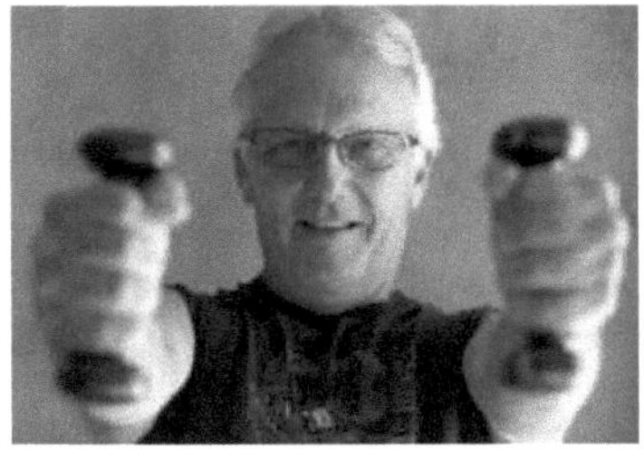

5. Calf Raises:

Add leg work to your routine and you'll be able to walk easier and farther. For the calf raise, stand 6-12 inches behind a sturdy chair with your feet hip-width apart. Hold on for balance. Inhale. Now, lift up high on your toes, exhaling slowly. Hold the raised position briefly. Lower your heels back to the ground, inhaling slowly. As you get stronger, do one leg at a time. Work up to two sets of 10-15 reps.

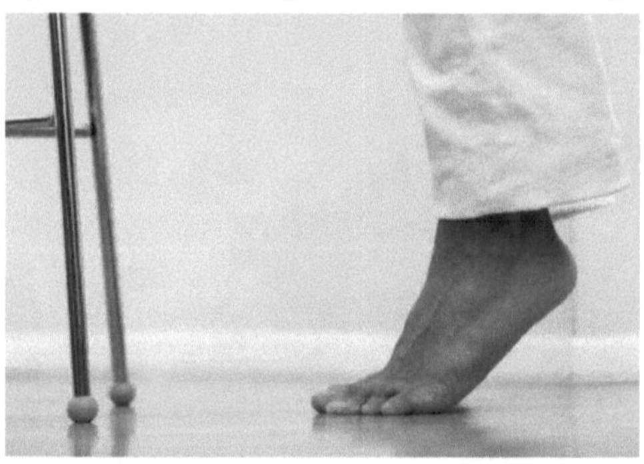

6. Leg Extensions:

For stronger thighs, sit in a chair that supports your back. Inhale. Now exhale slowly as you stretch one leg as straight as you can, without locking your knee. Breathe in as you slowly lower your foot back to the floor. Do one set with your right leg, then one set with your left. Getting too easy? Add ankle weights. Work up to two sets of 10-15 reps.

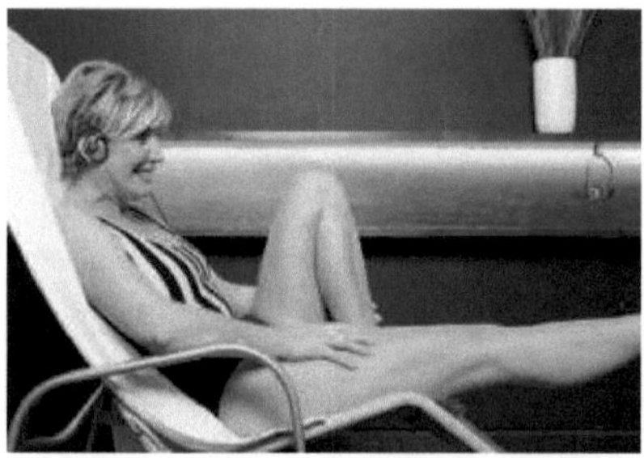

7. Exercise Your Diaphragm

This move strengthens a key breathing muscle, the diaphragm. Lie down with your knees bent or sit in an easy chair -- one hand on your chest, one below your rib cage. Slowly inhale through your nose so that your stomach raises one hand. Exhale with pursed lips and tighten your stomach. The hand on your chest should not move. Do this for 5 to 10 minutes, three or four times a day. Breathing this way will become easy and automatic.

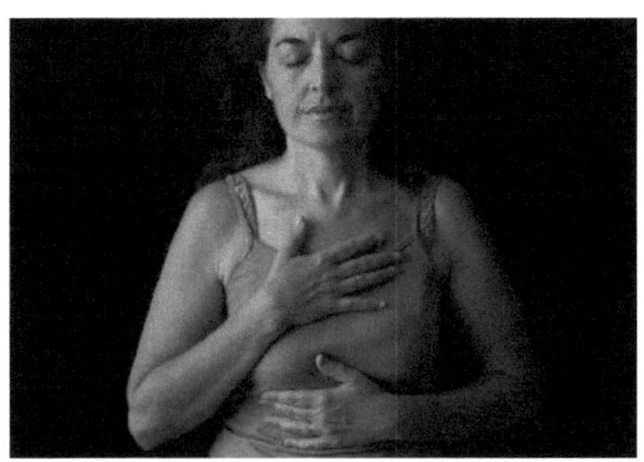

8. Chair Dance:

If you love to dance, try this armchair version in a class or with a DVD at home. Different programs can get your heart pumping, or pump up your muscles, or both -- to all kinds of music, from big band to hip hop. Beginners might start with a class to learn the safest ways to swing and bend. Adding hand weights can increase the challenge -- and your fitness level.

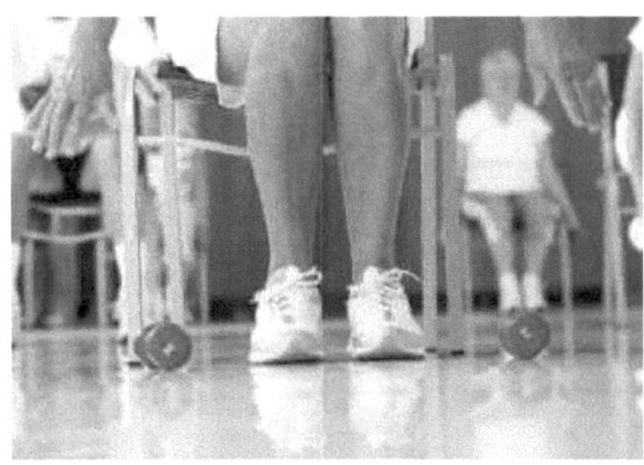

9. Breathe Right for Better Results

Breathe slowly during exercise. Inhale through your nose with your mouth closed. This warms and filters the air. Exhale through your mouth for twice as long as your inhale. Don't pant. That keeps your lungs from getting all the air out.

If your breath gets fast or shallow, stop and rest. Relax your body. Do pursed lip breathing: in through the nose and out slowly through pursed lips.

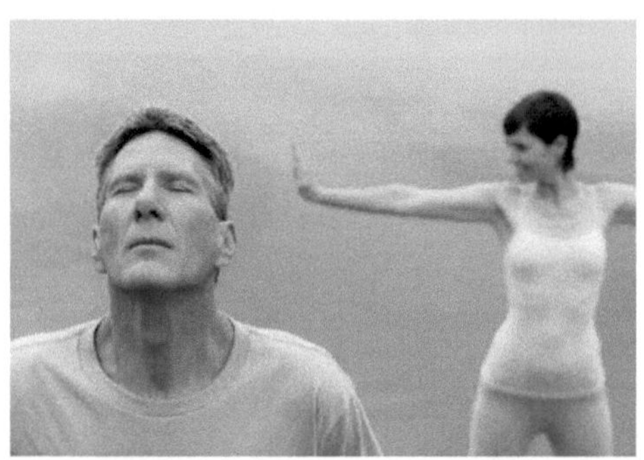

10. Schedule a Stretch:

Stretch gently before and after a workout. One stretch to try: Put your hands flat on a wall at arm's length and shoulder height. Step forward and bend your right knee. Bend your left knee until you feel a slight stretch in your calf. It shouldn't hurt. Hold for 10 to 30 seconds and repeat with left leg. Continue switching legs for three to five reps on each leg.

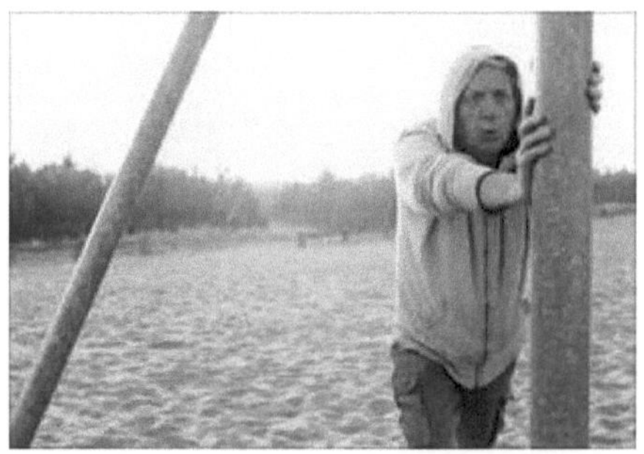

11. Try a New Way to Move

Jogging, skating, or rowing can be good exercises for people with mild COPD -- and fun ways to avoid workout boredom. Some activities do double duty, like water aerobics, which is good for COPD and arthritis. For beginners, a pulmonary rehab program is a good, safe place to start. Some people may need to avoid push-ups, sit-ups, or heavy lifting. Ask your doctor what's right for you.

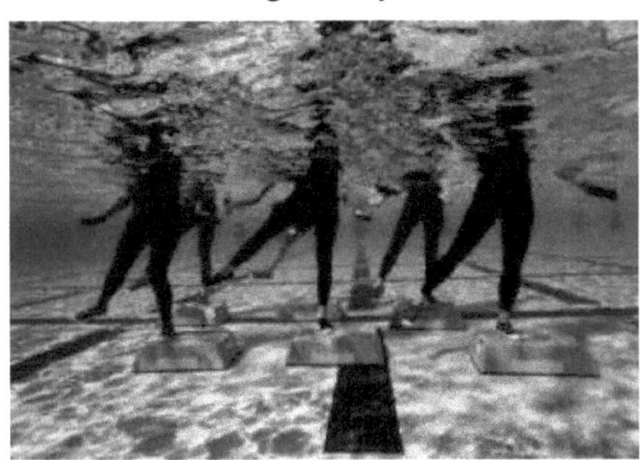

12. Exercising on Oxygen

If you use oxygen, you may worry that the equipment will be a hazard or a hassle. But if your doctor says to use oxygen during exercise, do it.

Extra-long tubing can help at home. Small, light-weight "travel" tanks keep you mobile. You can do most exercises with oxygen.

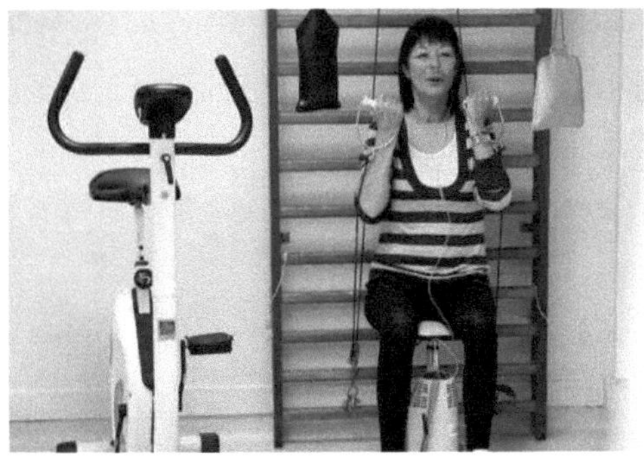

13. When Not to Exercise:

Give yourself a day off if your COPD symptoms are acting up: you're wheezing, coughing up more fluids than usual, or are unusually short of breath. You may want to talk to your doctor. Call for help right away for shortness of breath that doesn't improve, fast or irregular heartbeat, and feeling dizzy or lightheaded.

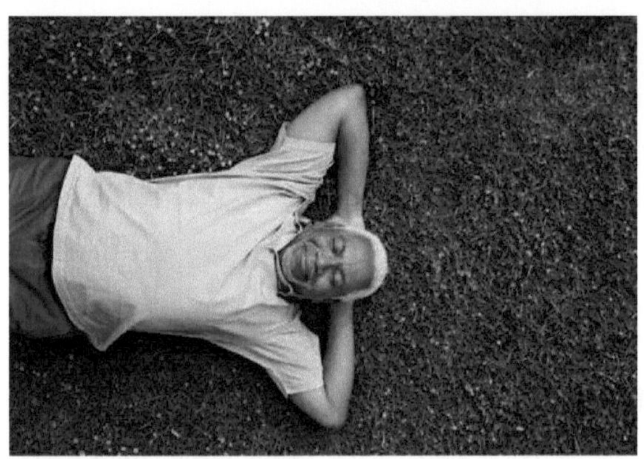

14. Make Exercise a Habit:

The goal for most people is to exercise for 20 to 30 minutes, at least three times a week. Include cardio and strength training. If you're out of shape, start a level that's comfortable -- even if it's just one minute. Ways to stay motivated include:

•Find an exercise buddy.

•Plan exercise in your daily routine.

•Keep an exercise journal -- and make notes as you feel better in your daily activities.

15. Stair climbing

- Hold the handrail lightly to keep your balance and to help yourself climb.
- Take your time.
- Step up while exhaling or breathing out with pursed lips. Place your whole foot flat on each step. Go up two steps with each exhalation.

- Inhale or breathe in while taking a rest before the next step.
- Going downstairs is much easier. Hold the handrail and place each foot flat on the step. Count the number of steps you take while inhaling, and take twice as many steps while exhaling.

16. Pursed-Lip Breathing for COPD:

This breathing exercise prevents air from being trapped in your lungs if you have COPD. Pursed-lip breathing allows you to breathe in more fresh air and reduces the anxiety and stress you may have from feeling short of breath. This is how it's done:

•Let your neck and shoulders relax.

•Breathe in through your nose while counting to three.

•Release all the air through your lips — purse your lips as though you were going to whistle.

•Exhale for twice as long as you inhaled, but don't force the air out.

"Pursed lip breathing is like smelling roses and blowing out a candle," explains Dr. Sochanski.

17. Diaphragmatic Breathing for COPD:

This breathing exercise for COPD patients helps strengthen your diaphragm, which is the dome-shaped muscle beneath your lungs that moves up and down as you breathe. With practice you should be able to get up to 12 deep breaths without tiring:

- Lie on your back with a pillow under your knees.
- Put one hand on your stomach and the other on your chest.
- As you breathe in, let your stomach rise, but try to keep your chest still.
- Breathe in to a count of three and then slowly breathe out through pursed lips to a count of six.

18. Deep Breathing for COPD

A lung health therapist can help you learn breathing exercises. "Once you learn them, you can do the exercises at home. Start slow and do the exercises at the same times each day," says Mardi Hayden, a respiratory therapist with the University of Connecticut Health Center in Farmington. "Find an exercise you like, and add more time as you get stronger. Always check with your doctor before starting any exercise program." COPD patients should practice deep breathing like this:

- Pull your elbows back firmly while standing or sitting.
- Take a deep breath.
- Hold it for the count of five.
- Exhale slowly and completely.

19. The Huff-Cough Technique for COPD

This exercise helps COPD patients cough more effectively without getting worn out. To practice this technique, follow these steps:

•While sitting in a chair, take several deep breaths as you would for diaphragmatic breathing.

•Place your hand over your stomach and breathe normally.

•Tighten up your stomach and chest muscles with your mouth open.

•Force air out while whispering the word "huff."

20. Exercises to avoid when you have COPD:

•Heavy lifting or pushing

•Chores such as shoveling, mowing, or raking

•Pushups, sit-ups, or isometric exercises, which involve pushing against immovable objects

•Outdoor exercises when the weather is very cold, hot, or humid

•Walking up steep hills

References:

A. Guz. (1991). The language of breathlessness: use of verbal descriptors by patients with cardiopulmonary disease. *Am. Rev. Respir. Dis.* 144:826–832.

Adams, L., and A. Guz. (1996). Lung Biology in Health and Disease, Vol. 90: Respiratory Sensation. Marcel Dekker, New York.

Alison B. & Kok P., (2003). A Simple Pulmonary Rehabilitation Program Improves Health Outcomes and Reduces Hospital Utilization in Patients with COPD, *CHEST,* 124.

Alison JA, Regnis JA, Donnelly PM, (1998). End-expiratory lung volume during arm and leg exercise in normal subjects and patients with cystic fibrosis. *Am J Respir Crit Care Med*, 158.

Altose, M., N. Cherniack, and A. P. Fishman. (1985). Respiratory sensations and dyspnea. *J. Appl. Physiol.* 58:1051–1054.

American College of Chest Physicians and American Association for Cardiovascular and Pulmonary Rehabilitation. Pulmonary rehabilitation: joint ACCP and AACVPR evidence-based guidelines. *Chest*, 1997;112(5):1363–96.

American Thoracic Society & European Respiratory Socity (2004). Standards for the diagnosis and management of patients with COPD, *Am Rev Respir Dis*, 2(4).

American Thoracic Society statement (2002). Guidelines for six minute walking test. *Am J Respir Crit Care Med*, 166.

American Thoracic Society, (1983). Screening for adult respiratory disease, *Am Rev Respir Dis*, 128.

American Thoracic Society, (1987). Standards for the diagnosis and care of patients with chronic obstructive pulmonary disease (COPD) and asthma. *Am Rev Respir Dis,* 136.

American Thoracic Society, (1999). Dyspnoea Mechanisms, Assessment, and Management: A Consensus Statement. *Am J Respir Crit Care Med*, 159.

American Thoracic Society, (2000). What constitutes an adverse health effect of air pollution. *Am J Respir Crit Care Med*, 161.

American Thoracic Society. (1995). Standards for the diagnosis and care of patients with chronic obstructive pulmonary disease. *Am. J.Respir. Crit. Care Med.* 152:S77–S120.

and symptom limitation in patients with chronic airflow limitation. *Am. Rev. Respir. Dis.* 146:935–940.

Anne E, Catherine J., (2004). Does Unsupported Upper Limb Exercise Training Improve Symptoms and Quality of Life for Patients With Chronic Obstructive Pulmonary Disease. *Journal of Cardiopulmonary Rehabilitation*, 24 (6).

Anthonisen NR, Connett JE, Kiley JP, (2010). Effects of smoking intervention and the use of an inhaled anticholinergic bronchodilator on the rate of decline of FEV1, The Lung Health Study JAMA, 272.

Astrand PO, Rodahl K, (1986). Textbook of work physiology. 3rd ed, New York, NY: McGraw-Hill.

Baarends E.M,. Schols A.M.W.J, Slebos D-J, Mostert R, Janssen P.P, Wouters E.F.M., (1995). Metabolic and ventilatory response pattern to arm elevation in patients with COPD and healthy age-matched subjects, *Eur Respir J*, 8.

Babcock MA, Pegelow DF, McLaran SR, (1995). Contribution of diaphragmatic power output to exercise-induced diaphragm fatigue, *J Appl Physiol*, 78.

Bauldoff, G. S., Hoffman, L. A., Sciurba, F., & Zullo, T. G., (1996). Home-based, upper-arm exercise training for patients with chronic obstructive pulmonary disease. Heart & Lung, *The Journal of Critical Care*, 25(4).

Beckerman, Marinella, Magadle, R. (2005). The Effects of 1 Year of Specific Inspiratory Muscle Training in Patients with COPD, *Chest*, 5.

Bellamy D, Bouchard J, Henrichsen S, Johansson G, (2006). International Primary Care Respiratory Group (IPCRG) Guidelines: Management of Chronic Obstructive Pulmonary Disease (COPD). *Prim Care Res Jou*, 15.

Belman MJ, Botnick WC, Shin JW. (1996). Inhaled bronchodilators reduce dynamic hyperinflation during exercise in patients with chronic obstructive pulmonary disease. *Am J Respir Crit Care Med*, 153.

Berger R, & Smith D. (2000). Effect of inhaled metaproterenol on exercise performance in patients with stable "fixed" airway obstruction. *Am Rev Respir Dis*, 138.

Bestall J C, Paul E A, Garrod R, Garnham R, Jones P W, Wedzicha J A., (1999). Usefulness of the Medical Research Council (MRC) dyspnoea scale as a measure of disability in patients with chronic obstructive pulmonary disease. *Thorax*, 54.

Black LF, Hyatt RE., (1969). Maximal respiratory pressures: normal values and the relationship to age and sex. *Am Rev Respir Dis*, 99.

Blackwell Scientific Publications, London.

Bolsher, D. C., B. G. Lindsey, and R. Shannon. (1987). Medullary inspiratory activity: influence of intercostal tendon organs and muscle spindle endings. *J. Appl. Physiol.* 62:1046–1056.

Bolsher, D. C., B. G. Lindsey, and R. Shannon. (1988). Respiratory pattern changes produced by intercostal muscle/rib vibration. *J. Appl. Physiol.* 84:1487–1491.

Bonnel A.M, Mathiot M.J, Grimaud C., (1985;). Inspiratory and Expiratory Resistive load Detection in Normal and Asthmatic Subjects. *Respiration*, 48.

Boutellier, U., and P. Piwko, (1992). The respiratory system as an exercise limiting factor in normal sedentary subjects. *Eur J Appl Physiol*, 64.

Breslin E H., (1992). The Pattern of Respiratory Muscle Recruitment during Pursed-Lip Breathing. *Chest*, 101.

Breslin E H., (1999). The Pattern of Respiratory Muscle Recruitment during Pursed-Lip Breathing. *Chest*, 101.

British Thoracic Society, (2001). Pulmonary rehabilitation, <u>Thorax</u>, 56.

Brusasco V. Pellegrino R. Rodarte J.R. (1997). Vital capacities in acute and chronic airway obstruction: dependence on flow and volume histories, *Eur Respir J*, 10.

BTS guidelines for the management of chronic obstructive pulmonary disease (1997). The COPDGuidelines Group of the Standards of Care Committee of the BTS. *Thorax*, 52(5).

Buist, A.S.; Vollmer, W.M.; McBurnie MA. (2008). World wide burden of COPD in high- and lowincome countries. Part I. The Burden of Obstructive Lung Disease (BOLD) Initiative. *Int. J. Tuberc. Lung Dis*, *12*, 703-708.

Burge P. S. (1999). Euroscop, Isolde and the Copenhagen City Lung Study. *Thorax*, 54.

Burt VL, Whelton P, Roccella EJ, (1995). Prevalence of hypertension in the US adult population: results from the Third National Health and Nutrition Examination Survey, 1988–1991, *Am Rev Respir Dis*, 25.

Campbell EJM, Freedman S, Smith PS, (1961). The ability of man to detect added elastic loads to breathing. *Clin Sci*, 20.

Carl-Peter Engstro¨m, Lars-Olof Persson, Sven Larsson and Marianne Sullivan, (1999). Long-Term Effects of a Pulmonary Rehabilitation Program in Outpatients with COPD: A Randomized Controlled Study, *Scand J Rehab Med*, 31.

Celli BR, MacNee W, (2004). Standards for the diagnosis and treatment of patients with COPD: a summary of the ATS/ERS position paper. *Eur Respir J*, 23.

Celli BR., (1994). The clinical use of upper extremity exercise. *Clin Chest Med*, 15.

Celli, B. R. (1995). Pulmonary rehabilitation in patients with COPD. *Am. J. Respir. Crit. Care Med*. 152:861–864.

Clanton TL, Dixon G, Drake J, Gadek JA., (1985). Inspiratory muscle conditioning using a threshold loading device, *Chest*, 96.

Coast JR, Clifford PS, Henrich TW, Stray-Gundersen J, Johnson RL. (1990). Maximal inspiratory pressure following maximal exercise in trained and untrained subjects. *Med Sci Sports Exerc*, 22 (6).

Corfield, D. R., G. R. Fink, S. C. Ramsay, K. Murphy, H. R. Harty, J. D. G. Watson, L. Adams, R. S. J. Frackowiak, and A. Guz. (1995). Evidence for limbic system activation during CO_2-stimulated breathing in man. *J. Physiol.* 488:77–84.

Couser J.I, Martinez F.J, Celli B.R., (1993). Pulmonary Rehabilitation That Includes Arm Exercise Reduces Metabolic and Ventilatory Requirements for Simple Arm Elevation. *Chest*, 103.

Covey K, Larson L, Wirtz E, Berry K, Pogue J, Alex G, Patel., (2001). High Intensity Inspiratory Muscle Training in Patients With Chronic Obstructive Pulmonary Disease and Severely Reduced Function, *Journal of Cardiopulmonary Rehabilitation*, 21.

Crapo RO, (1994).Pulmonary-function testing. *N Engl J Med*, 331.

Darlene & Baljit, (1995). Respiratory Muscle Training for Patients With Chronic Obstructive Pulmonary Disease, *Phys Ther*, 75.

Dekhuijzen PNR, Folgening HTM, van Herwaarden CLA., (1991). Target-flow inspiratory muscle training during pulmonary rehabilitation in patients with COPD. *Chest*, 99.

Devereux, (2006). ABC of chronic obstructive pulmonary disease Definition, epidemiology, and risk factors. *BMJ,* 332.

Dolmage E, Maestro, Monica A, Avendano, (1993). The Ventilatory Response to Arm Elevation of Patients With Chronic Obstructive Pulmonary Disease. *Chest*, 104.

Don D, Sin and Jack V. (2001). Inhaled Corticosteroids and the Risk of Mortality and Readmission In Elderly Patients with Chronic Obstructive Pulmonary Disease. *Am J Respir Crit Care Med*, 164.

Donner C.F, Muir J.F. (1997). Selection criteria and programmes for pulmonary rehabilitation in COPD patients. *Eur Respir J,*10.

Eagan TM, Gulsvik A, Eide GE, Bakke PS, (2004).Remission of respiratory symptoms by smoking and occupational exposure in a cohort study. *Eur Respir J*, 23.

Eastwood PR, Hillman DR, Morton AR, (1998). The effect oflearning on the ventilatory responses to inspiratory thresholdloading. *Am J Respir Crit Care Med*, 158.

Enright, S. J., Unnithan, Viswanath B., Heward, C., Withnall, L., Davies, David H. (2006). Effect of High-Intensity Inspiratory Muscle Training on Lung Volumes, Diaphragm Thickness, and Exercise Capacity in Subjects Who Are Healthy, *Physical Therapy*, 86.

Enright, S., Chatham, K., Lonescu, A. (2004). Inspiratory Muscle Training Improves Lung Function and Exercise Capacity in Adults with Cystic Fibrosis, *Chest*, 2.

Ezzati M, Lopez AD.(2012). Estimates of global mortality attributable to smoking in 2011. *Lancet*, 362.

Fatma A.M, (2012). Does Inspiratory Muscle Training Following Thoracic Surgery Have an Effect On The Outcomes? *Journal of American Science*, 8(3).

Fishman, A. P. (1994). NIH workshop summary: pulmonary rehabilitation research. *Am. J. Respir. Crit. Care Med.* 149:825–833.

Folgering H. Rooyackers J., (1998). Pulmonary rehabilitation in chronic obstructive pulmonary disease, *Eur Respir J*, 11.

Francisco, O. Javier, T. Pilar, C. (2002). Comparison of Effects of Strength and Endurance Training in Patients with Chronic Obstructive Pulmonary Disease, *Am J Respir Crit Care Med*, 166.

Gallagher CG. (1994). Exercise limitation and clinical exercise testing in chronic obstructive pulmonary disease. *Clin Chest Med*, 15:305–26.

Geddes EL, Reid WD, Crowe J, O'Brien K, Brooks D. (2005). Inspiratory muscle training in adults with chronic obstructive pulmonary disease: A systematic review, *Respir Med*, 99.

Gibala, M.J., J.P. Little, M. van Essen, G.P. Wilkin, K.A. Burgomaster, A. Safdar, S. Raha, and M.A. Tarnopolsky (2006). Short-term sprint interval versus traditional endurance training: similar initial adaptations in human skeletal muscle and exercise performance. *J. Physiol,* 57(3).

Gigliotti F, Coli C, Bianchi R, (2003). Exercise training improves exertional dyspnoea in patients with COPD: evidence of role of mechanical factors. *Chest*, 123.

Gigliotti F, Coli C, Bianchi R, (2005). Arm exercise and hyperinflation in patients with COPD, Effect of arm training, *Chest*, 128.

Global Initiative for Chronic Obstructive Pulmonary Lung Disease, (2011). Pocket Guide to COPD Diagnosis, Management, and Prevention, USA.

Global Strategy for the Diagnosis, Management and Prevention of COPD. Global Initiative for Chronic Obstructive Lung Disease (GOLD) 2008.

Goldstein R, De Rosie J, Long S, Dolmage T and Avendano M A., (1989). Applicability of a Threshold Loading Device for Inspiratory Muscle Testing and Training in Patients with COPD. *Chest* 96.

Gorman, J. M., M. R. Fyer, R. Goetz, J. Askanazi, M. R. Leibowitz, A. J. Fyer, J. Kinney, and D. F. Klein. (1988). Ventilatory physiology of patients with panic disorder. *Arch. Gen. Psychiatry* 45:31–39.

Gosselink R, Troosters T and Decramer M (1996). Peripheral muscle weakness contributes to exercise limitation in COPD, *American Journal of Respiratory and Critical Care Medicine*, 153.

Guz, A. (1997). Brain, breathing and breathlessness. *Respir. Physiol.* 109:197–204.

Haccoun C, Smountas AA, Gibbons WJ, Bourbeau J, Lands LC. (2002). Isokinetic muscle function in COPD. *Chest*, 121:1079–84.

Halbert, R.J.; Natoli, J.L.; Gano, A.; Badamgarav, E.; Buist, A.S.; Mannino, D.M. (2008). Global burden of COPD: systematic review and meta-analysis. *Eur. Respir. J*, 28, 523-532.

Hamilton AL, Killian KJ, Summers E and Jones NL (1995). Muscle strength, symptom intensity, and exercise capacity in patients with cardiorespiratory disorders, *American Journal of Respiratory and Critical Care Medicine*, 152.

Harver A, Mahler DA, Daubenspeck JA., (1989). Targeted inspiratory muscle training improves respiratory muscle function and reduces dyspnea in patients with COPD, *Ann Intern Med*, 111.

Hasford B, Fruhmann G. (1998). Air pollution and daily admissions for chronic obstructive pulmonary disease in six European cities: results from the APHEA project. Air pollution and Health, European Approach, *Eur Respir J*, 11.

Hay JG, Stone P, Carter J, (1998). Bronchodilator reversibility, exercise performance and breathlessness in stable chronic obstructive pulmonary disease. *Eur Respir J*, 5.

Hildegard SR, Rubio TM, Ruiz FO, (2001). Inspiratory muscle training in patients with COPD, *Chest*, 120.

Hill, Jenkins, Hillman, (2004). Dyspnoea in COPD: Can inspiratory muscle training help. *Aust Jour of Phy*, 50.

Howell, J. B. L., and E. J. M. Campbell, editors. (1966). Breathlessness.

John F, Jay A, Robert J, Homer A. (2000). Textbook of respiratory medicine, WB. Saunders company, 3.

Kikuchi, Y., S. Okabe, G. Tamura, W. Hida, M. Homma, K. Shirato, and T. Takishima. (1994). Chemosensitivity and perception of dyspnea in patients with a history of near-fatal asthma. *N. Engl. J. Med.* 330: 1329–1334.

Killian KJ, LeBlanc P, Martin DH, Summers E, Jones NL, Campbell EJ. (1992). Exercise capacity and ventilatory, circulatory, and symptom limitation in patients with chronic airflow limitation. *Am Rev Respir Disord,* 146:935–40.

Killian, K. J., E. Summers, N. L. Jones, and E. J. M. Campbell. (1992). Dyspnea and leg effort during incremental cycle ergometry. *Am. Rev. Respir. Dis.* 145:1339–1345.

Ko, F.W.S.; Hui, D.S.C.; Lai, C.K.W. (2008). Worldwide burden of COPD in high- and low-income countries. Part III. Asia-Pacific studies. *Int. J. Tuberc. Lung Dis. 12*, 713-717.

Koppers J. H, Vos J. E, Boot R. L, and Folgering M. (2006). Exercise Performance Improves in Patients With COPD due to Respiratory Muscle Endurance Training. *Chest*, 129.

Koulouris N.G. Rapakoulias P. Rassidakis A. Dimitroulis J. Gaga M. Milic-Emili J. Jordanoglou J. (1997). Dependence of forced vital capacity manoeuvre on time course of preceding inspiration in patients with restrictive lung disease, *Eur Respir J*, 10.

Lacasse Y, Brosseau L, Milne S, Martin S, Wong E, Guyatt GH, Goldstein RS. (2006). Pulmonary rehabilitation for chronic obstructive pulmonary disease. *Cochrane Database Syst Rev*, 3.

Lacasse Y, Rousseau L, Maltais F. (2001). Prevalence of depressive symptoms and depression in patients with severe oxygen-dependent chronic obstructive pulmonary disease. *J Cardiopulm Rehabil*, 20:80–86.

Larson JL, Kim h1J. Sharp JT, Larson DA. (1988). Inspiratory muscle training with a pressure threshold breathing device in patients with chronic obstructive pulmonary disease. *Am Rer, Respir Dis*, 138.

Larson JL, Kim MJ, Sharp JT, Larson DA. (1986). Inspiratory muscle training with a pressure threshold breathing device in patients with chronic obstructive pulmonary disease (abstract). *Am Rev Resp Dis*, 133.

Laurell CB, Eriksson S. (1963).The electrophoretic a1-globulin pattern of serum in a1-antitrypsin deficiency. *Scand J Clin Lab Invest*, 15.

Lausted, C.; Johnson, A.; Scott, W.; Johnson, M.; Coyne, K.; Coursey, D. (2006). Maximum static inspiratory and expiratory pressures with different lung volumes, *Biomedical engineering online*,5(1).

Leith DE, Mead J. (1967). Mechanisms determining residual volume of the lungs in COPD patients. *J Appl Physiol*, 23.

Lisboa C, Villafranca C, Leiva A, (1997). Inspiratory muscle training in chronic airflow limitation: effect on exercise performance, *Eur Respir J*, 10.

Lisboa C. Muñoz V. Beroiza T. Leiva A. Cruz E., (1994). Inspiratory muscle training in chronic airflow limitation: comparison of two different training loads with a threshold device, *Eur Respir J*, 7.

Lomax, (2010). Inspiratory muscle training, altitude, and arterial oxygen desaturation: a preliminary investigation, *Aviat Space Environ Med*, 81(5).

Manning H.L and Mahler D.A., (2001). Pathophysiology of dyspnoea. *Monaldi Arch Chest Dis*, 56: 4.

Manning, H. L., and R. M. Schwartzstein. (1995). Pathophysiology of dyspnea. *N. Engl. J. Med.* 333:1547–1553.

Mannino DM. (2002). COPD: epidemiology, prevalence, morbidity, mortality, and disease heterogeneity. *Chest*, 121 Suppl 5:121–26S.

Mannino, D.M.; Buist, A.S. (2007). Global burden of COPD: risk factors, prevalence, and future trends. *Lancet, 370*, 765-773.

Marco F. Di, Milic-Emili J, Boveri B, Carlucci P, Santus P, Casanova F, Cazzolaz M, Centanni S. (2003). Effect of inhaled bronchodilators on inspiratory capacity and dyspnoea at rest in COPD. <u>Eur Respir J</u>, 21.

Marsh, S.; Aldington, S.; Shirtcliffe, P.; Weatherall, M.; Beasley, R. (2006). Smoking and COPD: what really are the risks? *Eur. Respir. J. 28*, 883-886.

Marshall R, Stone R.W, Christie R.V., (1954). The Relationship of Dyspnoea to Respiratory Effort in Normal Subjects, Mitral Stenosis and Emphysema, *Clin.Ris, 13*.

Martinez FJ, Vogel PD, Dupont DN, (1993). Supported arm exercise vs unsupported arm exercise in the rehabilitation of patients with severe chronic airflow obstruction. *Chest*, 103.

McKeough ZJ, Alison JA and Bye PTB, (2003). Arm positioning alters lung volumes in subjects with COPD and healthy subjects. *Aust Jour of Phys,* 49.

Menezes, A.M.B.; Perez-Padilla, R.; Hallal, P.C.; Jardim, J.R.; Muiño, A.; Lopez, M.V.; Valdivia, G.; Pertuze, J.; Montes, de Oca M.; Tálamo, C. for the PLATINO Team. (2008). Worldwide burden of COPD in high- and low-income countries. Part II. Burden of chronic obstructive lung disease in Latin America: the PLATINO study. *Int. J. Tuberc. Lung Dis. 12*,709-712.

Morrison N J, Richardson J, Dunn L and Pardy R L. (1989). Respiratory Muscle Performance in Normal Elderly Subjects and Patients with COPD. *Chest*, 95.

Needham M and Stockley A.R. (2004). A1-Antitrypsin deficiency. 3: Clinical manifestations and natural history. *Thorax,* 59.

Newall, C. Stockley R A. & Hill S L., (2005). Exercise training and inspiratory muscle training in patients with COPD, *Thorax*, 60.

Nici L. (2000). Mechanisms and measures of exercise intolerance in chronic obstructive pulmonary disease. *Clin Chest Med*, 21(4):693–704.

Noseda A, Carpiaux J-P, Schmerber J, Valente F, Yernault J-C., (1994). Dyspnoea and flow-volume curve during exercise in COPD patients. *Eur Respir J*, 7.

O'Donnell DE, Webb KA., (1993). Exertional breathlessness in patients with chronic airflow limitation: the role of lung hyperinflation, *Am Rev Respir Dis*, 148.

Oga T, Nishimura K, Tsukino M, Sato S, Hajiro T. (2003). Analysis of the factors related to mortality in chronic obstructive pulmonary disease: role of exercise capacity and health status. *Am J Respir Crit Care Med*,167:544–49.

Paltiel W, Rasmi M, Marinella B, Margalit W, and Noa Berar-Yanay, (2003). Specific Expiratory Muscle Training in COPD, *CHEST*, 124.

Potter WA, Olafsson S, Hyatt R, (1971). Ventilatory mechanicsand expiratory flow limitation during exercise in patients with obstructive lung disease, *Chest*, 50.

Preusser BA, Winningham ML, Clanton TL. (1994). High- vs low-intensity inspiratory muscle interval training in patients with COPD, *Chest*, 106.

Q. Hamid, J. Shannon and J. Martin (2006). Physiologic Basis of Respiratory Disease. BC Decker Inc., Hamilton, Ontario, Canada, *European Respiratory Journal*. 1-793.

Quanjer PhH, Tammeling GJ, Cotes JE, Pedersen OF, Peslin R, Yernault J-C. (1993). Lung volumes and forced ventilator flows. Report Working Party, "Standardization of Lung Function Tests". European Coal and Steel Community. Official statement of the European Respiratory Society. *Eur Respir J*, 6(16).

Ramirez-Venegas A, Sansores RH, Perez-Padilla R et al., (2006).Survival of patients with chronic obstructive pulmonary disease due to biomass smoke and tobacco. <u>Am J Respir Crit Care Med</u>, 173.

Reid W and Dechman, (1995). Considerations When Testing and Training the Respiratory Muscles. *Phys ther*, 75.

Reilly JJ, Silverman EK, Shapiro S. D, Favoi AS, et al., (2008).Chronic Obstructive Pulmonary Disease. In: Harrison's Principles of Internal Medicine. *Mc Graw Hill Medical*: New York. 2(17).

Ribarren C, Tekawa IS, Sidney S, Friedman GD. (1999).Effect of cigar smoking on the risk of cardiovascular disease, chronic obstructive pulmonary disease, and cancer in men. *N Engl J Med*, 340.

Richardson RS, Sheldon J, Poole DC, Hopkins SR, Ries AL, Wagner PD. (1999). Evidence of skeletal muscle metabolic reserve during whole body exercise in patients with chronic obstructive pulmonary disease. *Am J Respir Crit Care Med*, 159:881–85.

Ries AL, Bauldoff GS, Carlin BW, (2007). Pulmonary Rehabilitation: Joint ACCP/ AACVPR Evidence-Based Clinical Practice Guidelines. *Chest*, 131.

Ries AL, Kaplan RM, Myers R, (2003). Maintenance after pulmonary rehabilitation in chronic lung disease: a randomised trial. *Am J Crit Care Respir Med*, 167.

Robert A. Wise, (2006). The Value of Forced Expiratory Volume in 1 Second Decline in the Assessment of Chronic Obstructive Pulmonary Disease Progression, *The American Journal of Medicine*, 119:(10).

Scherer A, Spengler M, Owassaplan, Imhof, Boutellier, (2000). Respiratory Muscle Endurance Training in Chronic Obstructive Pulmonary Disease Impact on Exercise Capacity, Dyspnoea, and Quality of Life. *Am J Respir Crit Care Med*, 162.

Schikowski T, Sugiri D, Ranft U (2005). Long-term air pollution exposure and living close to busy roads are associated with COPD in women. *Respir Res*, 6.

Schwartzstein, R. M. (1998). The language of dyspnea. *In* D. A. Mahler, editor. Lung Biology in Health and Disease, Vol. 111: Dyspnea. Marcel Dekker, New York. 35–62.

Schwartzstein, R. M., and L. M. Cristiano. (1996). Qualities of respiratory sensation. *In* L. Adams and A. Guz, editors. Lung Biology in Health and Disease, Vol. 90: Respiratory Sensation. Marcel Dekker, New York. 125–154.

Sciurba F, Criner GJ, Lee SM, Mohsenifar Z, Shade D, Slivka W (2003). Six-minute walk distance in chronic obstructive pulmonary disease: reproducibility and effect of walking course layout and length. *Am. J Respir. Crit Care Med*, 167.

Scott K, Bartolome R, Fernando J, James I, Jairo MD, (1997). Arm Training Reduces the VO2 and VE Cost of Unsupported Arm Exercise and Elevation in Chronic Obstructive Pulmonary Disease. *Journal of Cardiopulmonary Rehabilitation*, 17 (3).

Serón P, Riedemann P, Muñoz S, Doussoulin A, Villarroel P, Cea X, (2005). Effect of Inspiratory Muscle Training on Muscle Strength and Quality of Life in Patients With Chronic Airflow Limitation: a Randomized Controlled Trial, *Arch Bronconeumol*, (11) 41.

Shad Ali, Deepak Talwar and S.K. Jain, (2014). The Effect of a Short-Term Pulmonary Rehabilitation on Exercise Capacity and Quality of Life in Patients Hospitalised with Acute Exacerbation of Chronic Obstructive Pulmonary Disease, *Indian J Chest Dis Allied Sci*, 56.

Shaffer, (2012). Effect of exercise training in patients with chronic obstructive pulmonary disease compared with healthy elderly subjects, *J Cardiopulm Rehabil Prev*, 32(3).

Shahin, Germain, Kazem, Annat, (2008). Benefits of short inspiratory muscle trainingon exercise capacity, dyspnea, and inspiratory fraction in COPD patients. *International Journal of COPD*, 3(3).

Sharp, J.T.J. Danon, W.S. Druz, N.B. Goldberg, H.C. fishman ,and W.Machnach, (1974). Respiratory muscle function in patients with chronic obstructive pulmonary disease :Its relationship to disability and to respiratory therapy. *Am Rev Respir Dis*, 110(1).

Shim C, Stover DE, Williams MH. (1978). Response to corticosteroids in chronic bronchitis. *J Allergy Clin Immunol*, 62.

Siafakas, N.M. Vermeire, P. Pride, N.B. (1995). Optimal assessment and management of chronic obstructive pulmonary disease (COPD), *Eur Respir J*, 8.

Simon, P. M., R. M. Schwartzstein, J. W. Weiss, K. LaHive, V. Fencl, M. Teghtsoonian, and S. E. Weinberger. (1989). Distinguishable sensations of breathlessness in normal volunteers. *Am. Rev. Respir. Dis.* 140:1021–1027.

Simon, P. M., R. M. Schwartzstein, J. W. Weiss, V. Fencl, M. Teghtsoonian, and S. E. Weinberger. 1990. Distinguishable types of dyspnea in patients with shortness of breath. *Am. Rev. Respir. Dis.* 142:

Smith K, Cook D, Guyatt GH, Madhavan J, Oxman AD. (1992). Respiratory muscle training in chronic airflow limitation: a meta-analysis. *Am Rev Respir Dis,* 145.

Soguel SN, Burdet L, de Muralt B, Fitting JW. (1996). Oxygen saturation during daily activities in chronic obstructive pulmonary disease. *Eur.Respir.J.* 9.

Solway S, Brooks D, Lau L and Goldstein RS., (2002). The short term effect of a collator on functional exercise capacity among individuals with severe COPD, *Chest,* 122.

Spruit M.A, Gosselink R, Troosters T, De Paepe K, Decramer M. (2002) Resistance versus endurance training in patients with COPD and peripheral muscle weakness. *Eur Respir J,* 19.

Sturdy, Hillman, Green, Jenkins, Cecins and Eastwood, (2003). Feasibility of High-Intensity, Interval-Based Respiratory Muscle Training in COPD. *Chest,* 123.

Sudo E, Ohga E, Matsuse T, Teramoto S, (1997). The effects of pulmonary rehabilitation combined with inspiratory muscle training on pulmonary function and inspiratory muscle strength in elderly patients with chronic obstructive pulmonary disease, *Nihon Ronen Igakkai Zasshi,* 34(11).

Suzuki S, Sato M, Okubo T. (1995). Expiratory muscle training and sensation of respiratory effort during exercise in normal subjects, *Thorax,* 50(4).

Swanney MP, Ruppel G, Enright PL, (2008). Using the lower limit of normal for the FEV1/FVC ratio reduces the misclassification of airway obstruction, *Thorax,* 63(12).

Takahashi, Jenkins, Geoffrey R, Watson P, (2003). A New Unsupported Upper Limb Exercise Test for Patients With Chronic Obstructive Pulmonary Disease. *Journal of Cardiopulmonary Rehabilitation,* 23.

Thierry, Richard, Rik, and Marc, (2005). Pulmonary Rehabilitation in Chronic Obstructive Pulmonary Disease, *Am J Respir Crit Care Med,* 172.

Thomas A. Scherer, Christina M. (2000). Respiratory Muscle Endurance Training in Chronic Obstructive Pulmonary Disease, Impact on Exercise Capacity, Dyspnea, and Quality of Life, *Am J Respir Crit Care Med,* 162.

Troosters T, Gosselink R, Decramer M. (1968). Six-minute walk test: a valuable test to measure physical ability. *Phys.Ther,* 32.

Troosters, T., Gosselink, R., Langer, D., & Decramer, M, (2007). Pulmonary rehabilitation in chronic obstructive pulmonary disease. *Respiratory Medicine: COPD,* 3(2).

Vanessa, & Carolina, (2011). Effects of inspiratory muscle training in COPD patients, *Elsevier Journal,* 33(1).

Vathenen AS, Britton JR, Ebden P, (1988). High-dose inhaled albuterol in severe chronic airflow limitation. *Am Rev Respir Dis,* 138.

Velloso, Stella, Cendon Silva, Jardim, (2003). Metabolic and Ventilatory Parameters of Four Activities of Daily Living Accomplished With Arms in COPD Patients. *Chest,* 123.

Vestbob, J. Sorensen, T. Lange, P. Brix, A. Torre, P. and Viskum, K. (1999). Long-term effect of inhaled budesonide in mild and moderate chronic obstructive pulmonary disease: a randomized controlled trial. *Lancet,* 353.

Villafranca, C. Borzone, G. Leiva, A. Lisboa C. (2010). Effect of inspiratory muscle training with an intermediate load on inspiratory power output in COPD, *Eur Respir J,* 11.

Volianitis, S. McConnell, A.K. Jones, D.A. (2005). Assessment of maximum inspiratory pressure (PImax): prior submaximal respiratory muscle activity ('warm-up') enhances PImax and attenuates the learning effect of repeated measurement, *Journal of Cardiopulmonary Rehabilitation,* 28.

Wanger JS, Ikle DN, Cherniack RM. (1996). The effect of inspiratory maneuvers on expiratory flow rates in health and asthma: influence of lung elastic recoil. *Am J Respir Crit Care Med,* 153.

Wasserman, K., and R. Cassaburi. (1988). Dyspnea: physiological and pathophysiological mechanisms. *Ann. Rev. Med.* 39:503–515.

Weiner P, Azgad Y and Ganam R. (1992). Inspiratory Muscle Training Combined with General Exercise Reconditioning in Patients with COPD. *Chest* 102.

Widdicombe, J. G. (1982). Pulmonary and respiratory tract receptors. *J. Exp. Biol.* 100:41–57.

William E. & Terry L. (2001). The Effects of Respiratory Muscle Training On Maximal and Submaximal Cardiovascular And Pulmonary Measurements, *Eur Respir J*, 11.

Wilson SH. Cooke NT. Edwards RHT. Spiro SG, (1984). Predicted normal values for maximal respiratory pressures in caucasian adults and children, *Thorax*, 39.

Wright, G. W., and B. V. Branscomb. (1954). Origin of the sensations of dyspnea. *Trans. Am. Clin. Climatol. Assoc.* 1966:116–125.

Younes, M. (1995). Mechanisms of respiratory load compensation. *In* J. A. Dempsey and A. L. Pack, editors. Regulation of Breathing, 2nd. Marcel Dekker, New York. 867–922.

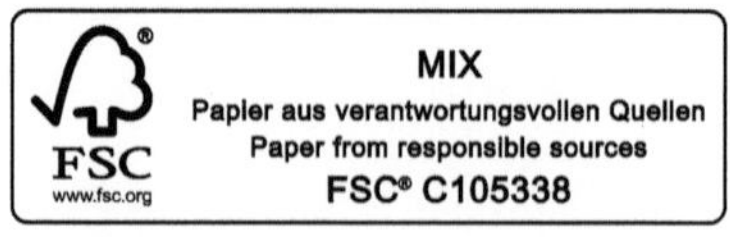

Printed by Books on Demand GmbH, Norderstedt / Germany